Routledge Revivals

Prospects for the National Health

The British National Health Service celebrated its thirtieth birthday in 1978. A Royal Commission was set up to consider the role of the National Health Service, and it is the debates that surrounded this Royal Commission that form the basis for the twelve topics covered by this book.

The economic difficulties that the country was facing when this book was published in 1979 highlighted the widely publicised malaise in the health service, and exposed the limitation of a set of ideals developed by the NHS in the years after the Second World War. These limitations, reflected in the economic recession of all industrial countries, presented a challenge and thus an opportunity to re-examine the nature and purpose of our health service.

Although this work offered no easy solutions, it did present significant implications for public debate and public appraisal of the prospects of the National Health Service, and greatly mirrors the debates that have been stirring in more recent years. This title will be of interest to students of sociology.

Prospects for the National Health

Edited by
Paul Atkinson
Robert Dingwall
Anne Murcott

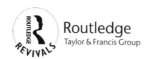

Routledge
Taylor & Francis Group

First published in 1979
by Croom Helm

This edition first published in 2016 by Routledge
2 Park Square, Milton Park, Abingdon, Oxon, OX14 4RN
and by Routledge
711 Third Avenue, New York, NY 10017

Routledge is an imprint of the Taylor & Francis Group, an informa business

© 1979 This edition. Introduction, selection, editorial matter Paul Atkinson,
Robert Dingwall and Anne Murcott. © Robert Dingwall Ch. 1. © Anne
Murcott Ch. 2. © Celia Davies Ch. 3. © Paul Atkinson Ch. 4. © Muir Gray
and Max Blythe Ch. 5. © Margaret Miers Ch. 6. © Denis Gregory Ch. 7. ©
Jane Taylor Ch. 8. © Rita Austin Ch. 9. © Gail Eaton and Barbara Webb Ch.
10. © John Grigg Ch. 11. © Stuart Henry and David Robinson Ch. 12.

Publisher's Note
The publisher has gone to great lengths to ensure the quality of this reprint but
points out that some imperfections in the original copies may be apparent.

Disclaimer
The publisher has made every effort to trace copyright holders and welcomes
correspondence from those they have been unable to contact.

A Library of Congress record exists under LC control number: 80467880

ISBN 13: 978-1-138-95240-9 (hbk)
ISBN 13: 978-1-315-66763-8 (ebk)
ISBN 13: 978-1-138-95245-4 (pbk)

PROSPECTS FOR
THE NATIONAL HEALTH

**Edited by PAUL ATKINSON,
ROBERT DINGWALL and ANNE MURCOTT**

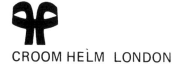

CROOM HELM LONDON

© 1979 This edition. Introduction, selection, editorial matter Paul Atkinson, Robert Dingwall and Anne Murcott. © Robert Dingwall Ch. 1. © Anne Murcott Ch. 2. © Celia Davies Ch. 3. © Paul Atkinson Ch. 4. © Muir Gray and Max Blythe Ch. 5. © Margaret Miers Ch. 6. © Denis Gregory Ch. 7. © Jane Taylor Ch. 8. © Rita Austin Ch. 9. © Gail Eaton and Barbara Webb Ch. 10. © John Grigg Ch. 11. © Stuart Henry and David Robinson Ch. 12.

Croom Helm Ltd, 2-10 St John's Road, London SW11

British Library Cataloguing in Publication Data

Prospects for the national health.
    1. Great Britain — National Health Service
    I. Atkinson, Paul   II. Dingwall, Robert
    III. Murcott, Anne
    362.1'0941   RA395.G6

    ISBN 0-85664-741-1

Printed and bound in Great Britain by
REDWOOD BURN LIMITED
Trowbridge & Esher

CONTENTS

INTRODUCTION

The British National Health Service is now thirty years old. Its birthday in 1978 found few willing to join in an unqualified celebration for, despite its outstanding achievements in improving the morbidity and mortality of a nation, many believe that it is in a state of 'crisis'. A Royal Commission has been set up 'to consider in the interests of the patients and of those who work in the National Health Service the best use and management of the financial and manpower resources of the National Health Service'. Whether or not one accepts the view that there is a crisis in the NHS, this is clearly a suitable time to take stock.

The debates surrounding the Royal Commission have prompted us to bring together this collection of essays on a number of central issues in the delivery of health care. We were concerned that the narrow emphasis on financial and manpower resources in the remit of the Royal Commission might lead to the neglect of more fundamental questions about the relationship between health and society. Only through debating such issues can informed judgements be reached as to the tasks which a health service could realistically be expected to assume; only through such debate can the consequences be appreciated for the forms of service delivery and for other institutions, such as personal social services, education, industry, families and neighbourhood communities.

The contributions have not been put together in an attempt to cover each and every aspect of the NHS: that would clearly have been a task beyond the scope of a single volume such as this. We believe, however, that our concentration on issues and problems will have a general relevance to any specific investigation. Although the majority of the authors are sociologists, we have tried to write for a general audience. The reader will find no 'party line'. Although there are common themes, each contributor speaks in his or her own right. This is not a manifesto or a blueprint for the future of the NHS, although important policy questions arise throughout the following chapters. This collection is intended to contribute to the debates which must precede such planning. In particular resource allocation and management can only be sensibly discussed after we have decided what is wanted from a health service. This decision is not a technical question for experts. It affects the way in which everyone lives — his or her plans, aspirations, and even dreams — and as such everyone has a part to play in making it.

The Nature of the Problem

We are not convinced that the supposed crisis of recent years is peculiar to the NHS. This is not to say that everything is in the best possible state. The recent, widely publicised malaise in the health service is real enough, at any rate in its consequences. As the press and television frequently remind us, wards lie empty for lack of staff, young babies are put at risk from shortages of equipment and trained personnel, old and unsuitable buildings continue to serve well beyond their proper structural life, long waiting lists persist for treatment of all kinds. Health workers are constantly faced by difficult and uncomfortable choices. Patients and their families continue to suffer pain and distress.

The source of these difficulties is not, however, the NHS itself, but rather the general economic climate in which it has been forced to operate. It has merely taken its share of the overall consequences of Britain's poor industrial performance. Capital spending has fallen victim to the uncertainties and expenses of 'stop-go' economic management. Health workers, from doctors to cleaners, have, like all public sector employees, borne the brunt of successive rounds of pay restraint. Given this lack of economic growth, expenditure on health care has not only risen slowly in absolute terms, but in relative terms growth has been restricted. We spend a lower proportion of our national income on health than do other industrialised countries including the United States, France and West Germany. There is, however, no direct relationship between the health of a country and its expenditure in that field. The USA, for example, spends about half as much again, in relative terms, on health care as does Britain. By almost any standard of morbidity and mortality, however, its population as a whole enjoys poorer health. Indeed it can be argued that Britain has enjoyed a remarkable bargain in the NHS.

As it exists today the NHS realises a set of ideals developed in the years after the Second World War. Our economic difficulties have exposed the limitations of those ideals, limitations which all industrialised countries are coming to recognise as the world slides into recession. The challenge is to respond positively to this crisis, to see it as an opportunity for a re-examination of the nature and purposes of health services rather than merely crying out for more of the same.

This Volume

The very title and designation of the National Health Service implies that it is, or should be, *national* in character, concerned with the *health* of the population and provides people with a *service*. In a common-sense way, of course, it is. The NHS is financed out of general taxation, is nationally available throughout the country and as a whole is ultimately accountable to Parliament. And to the extent that 'health', 'illness' and 'medicine' comprise a package of related concepts, it is all about health. But this common-sense view itself militates against the national health service that the NHS could be. There are underlying biases, ideologies and interests which perpetuate this kind of thinking, and which are perpetuated by it and which impede the realisation of a truly national health service.

Robert Dingwall (chapter 1) discusses some of the enduring features of the NHS which have tended towards the perpetuation of unequal access to health care and unequal incidence of morbidity and mortality. Although overall standards of health have improved, the inequalities of class and geography have changed little. As Dingwall reminds us, the NHS was not born of a desire for redistributive justice and it has continued to reflect prevailing social and economic differences. Aneurin Bevan said of the health service that it was 'conditioned and limited by the evils it was intended to remove' and its subsequent development has done little to modify that judgement. At the same time as underlining the persistence of inequality, Dingwall warns us against any oversimplified reaction to this 'failure' on the part of the NHS. Health services cannot compensate for society and the present form of the NHS reflects a particular set of political and moral choices. The biases are predicated on essentially ideological premises. Without a reappraisal of these choices the NHS, of itself, cannot be expected to bring about social changes.

These remarks are echoed by Anne Murcott (chapter 2) who stresses the essentially ideological nature of concepts of 'health'. It is widely remarked that the NHS has done little to foster 'health', on either a collective or individual basis, but has merely responded to 'sickness'. One of the clichés of debate in health care is that we have a National *Illness* Service rather than a National *Health* Service. Although some critics of the NHS, and health care in industrialised societies in general, advocate greater attention to preventive measures, a reorientation of priorities towards collective health is not a simple alternative. There is, indeed, a real danger of seeing curative medicine as ideologically tainted, while preventive and 'community' orientations are hailed as promoting 'health' as if this were unquestionably natural, unproblematic, and hence superior. But Murcott emphasises that 'health' is as much a matter of moral judgement as any other valued personal or social state of affairs, and must be examined just as critically. As Dingwall suggests, a society which maximised 'health' would not necessarily be the sort of society in which many people might wish to live.

An individualistic emphasis runs through the NHS, not least in the very models of sickness and medical practice which are enshrined in it. Dingwall's paper discusses the history of this approach, while Celia Davies (chapter 3) discusses its modern forms in her analysis of hospital-centred health care. This does not refer simply to the location of the service, but to a general and distinctive way of thinking about health problems. This includes, she argues, 'a curative rather than a preventive orientation, an individualistic, one-to-one service bias . . . a technological approach . . . a focus on acute and episodic rather than chronic illness'. It is a way of thinking which freezes the second of McKeown's (1971) three phases of the development of British medicine. In this thesis, during the first phase, up to about 1937, improvements in the general health of the nation derived from environmental and nutritional changes. The second stage, from 1937 to 1954, saw the development of many powerful new drugs and surgical techniques together with an 'engineering' model of treatment stressing specific procedures for specific therapeutic goals. This phase saw the origins of the NHS, but the succeeding years have served mainly to display the limitations of this model. The organisational and ideological structures of the NHS have, nevertheless, changed little. Paul Atkinson (chapter 4) shows one way in which they are reproduced through the hospital-centred pattern of medical education, which is, in turn, reflected in the collective and individual aspirations of the profession.

Recently there have, of course, been attempts to shift the emphasis of the NHS towards prevention, but these have taken place at a technical level with no real challenge to the underlying concepts of health and illness. The papers by Dingwall and Murcott touch on some of the consequent issues and this also forms the background to Muir Gray and Max Blythe's essay (chapter 5) on the failure of health education. While this area has enjoyed rapid expansion of late, many programmes in health education are still conceived solely as a 'response to the threat of illness' and lack any positive concept of health. Gray and Blythe retain a more optimistic view of the possibilities of health education than several other contributors, provided that it can be more adequately grounded in the culture of its target groups. The political and philosophical problems which arise must be respected but need not be allowed to undermine the whole enterprise.

Margaret Miers (chapter 6) and Denis Gregory (chapter 7) also highlight the need to re-examine notions of health. They stress how closely health and illness are interwoven with the patterns of production and consumption in contemporary industrial societies. Gregory indicates the shortcomings of current provision for occupational health care. The only answer, in his view, is to integrate occupational health services with the NHS, since health risks arise wherever people work. In the same way, well-established social customs may have serious consequences for health. We have come to think quite readily of smoking as one of these and, as Miers describes, the risks run by adolescents in their cars and on their motorbikes are part of contemporary life styles. She goes on to argue that even such long-established and cherished institutions as marriage can carry associated risks.

In the development of the NHS, Britain can be proud to have preserved a general practitioner service, but the price has been to make the provision of primary care almost exclusively *domestic* in character (the designation 'family practitioner' is revealing). While Gregory and Miers show the consequences of neglecting health risks in industrial and recreational settings, Jane Taylor (chapter 8) looks at some unacknowledged difficulties in the domestic situation. She gives a glimpse of the hidden labour involved in health care at home, depending on the unpaid efforts of family members. It is a timely caution against some of the more unthinking advocates of a shift from hospital-centred medicine to 'community care'. This latter is in serious danger of becoming merely a euphemism for further exploitation of a reserve army of (usually female) relatives, neighbours and friends. Because this labour is unpaid, it appears to have no cost, a feature no doubt seductive to the narrow financial mind. The NHS can effect savings without any consideration of even the economic costs to the nation as a whole, let alone the personal costs to morally blackmailed kin.

The allocation of work within the health service and between health and other personal services forms a final theme in this collection. The essays by Gregory and Atkinson already mentioned raise questions about the division of labour within the medical profession. Gregory looks for a greater emphasis on the provision of medical personnel to the industrial sector. Atkinson shows how debates over *numbers* of doctors involve a set of claims which direct us towards an examination of the division of labour between specialties as well as the vertical career structure in medicine.

Rita Austin (chapter 9) and Gail Eaton and Barbara Webb (chapter

10) consider the possible futures for two occupations — nursing and pharmacy. Both note the drive for professionalisation, the search for greater autonomy and clinical responsibility by these paramedical occupations. The authors' responses to this differ: Austin favours an enhanced role for the nurse practitioner, while Eaton and Webb have reservations about the ambitions of clinical pharmacy. The effect of these occupational claims is to challenge the dominance of the medical profession by encroaching on their traditional domain. The consequences of the professional status of medicine have frequently been criticised. Doctors are presented as self-appointed arbiters of health and medicine, arrogating the right to pass judgement on matters of private and public morality, and as having imperial ambitions towards the 'medicalisation' of everyday life. This thesis is not without its problems. Phil Strong (in press) has recently argued that the attack has much to do with the rival imperialism of sociology and, in some respects, is sharply at odds with the observable nature of medical practice. Nevertheless, in so far as the critics of medicalisation have a valid case, it is not at all evident that the professionalisation of other health workers is in the public interest. The realignments and redistributions discussed by Austin and by Eaton and Webb may reduce the dominance of the medical profession. There is, however, no guarantee that enhanced status in the future might not merely reproduce the more undesirable aspects of traditional medical dominance.

It seems apparent, on the other hand, that this dominance cannot in any case hope to survive in its present form. John Grigg's essay (chapter 11) examines the manner in which auxiliary workers and doctors each handle industrial disputes in the NHS. In seeking to ensure the maintenance of what they regard as adequate pay, status and working conditions, doctors have been increasingly drawn into the adoption of union tactics in their industrial relations. At the same time, such actions threaten to jeopardise their claimed allegiance to the proprieties of professionalism. If, in this way, their work loses something of its mystery, they must expect still greater pressures for public scrutiny of their activities.

Finally we come to consider relations between professional health workers and the lay community. We have already mentioned Taylor's analysis of the role of unpaid care in the health service. Stuart Henry and David Robinson (chapter 12) discuss the growth of self-help movements and their appeal to radicals and established interests alike. They criticise the naive romanticism of claims that this movement amounts to a popular reappropriation of health care. Many self-help groups, in fact, incorporate and celebrate professional medical perspectives; they may, indeed, even owe their existence to the encouragement of a segment of the medical profession. While they have a useful part to play they cannot be seen in simplistic, oppositional terms.

This book offers no easy answers, then. In so far as there is a common approach underlying the various essays, it is a distrust of utopian solutions. Whether the future leads in a more collectivist or a more individualist direction as a result of the Royal Commission, there will be costs as well as benefits. The relative balance of advantage is one which is of crucial importance to everyone. As such it is perhaps too important to abandon to experts, politicians, or the self-interest of professions merely because of the difficulty of the problems. It is our hope that this collection will contribute to a public debate and to a public appraisal of the prospects for the National Health.

The original idea for this volume came from Rita Austin, and the editors would like to acknowledge the very great part which she played in the planning stage. A change of job and the pressure of work meant that she was unable to maintain a close involvement with the book, but the final product still reflects much of her early work and owes a great deal to her. We should also like to thank Llewela Gibbons for her meticulous preparation of the typescript.

Since our aim in this volume was to address a wider audience than just fellow specialists, we urged the contributors to avoid burdening their papers with unnecessarily detailed references and footnotes. Since there was a good deal of duplication in the works cited we have consolidated the references into a single bibliography at the end of the volume.

1 INEQUALITY AND THE NATIONAL HEALTH SERVICE

Robert Dingwall

In recent years, there has been a substantial body of criticism of the National Health Service for its failure to remedy inequalities in the incidence of disease and premature death and in the distribution of health care. This criticism has come from both conservative and socialist commentators, using this alleged failure as a ground for proposing alternative solutions based on a greater adherence to principles either of individual responsibility or of collective regulation. In this paper, I intend to argue that such a charge is fundamentally mistaken and that the NHS has never had the promotion of equality in health as a particularly salient objective. The NHS, and other personal social services, are the product of a particular historical compromise between individual and collective rights and obligations and the 'crisis' in the Welfare State proclaimed from both critical positions is due to the exhaustion of the political movement which underwrote that compromise, British social democracy. Certain choices about the nature of our society cannot continue to be avoided by the Butskellite consensus on the respective roles of individualist and collectivist tendencies in social and economic policy. The choice between individualism and collectivism is not, however, an easy one to make and each route has its costs as well as its benefits.

Inequalities in Health

Although the purpose of this paper is to discuss some of the reasons why inequalities arise and persist in health and not to duplicate the work of others such as Townsend (1974), Blaxter (1976) or Hart (1978) in detailing the generally agreed facts of inequality in mortality and morbidity, it is, perhaps, worth reminding ourselves of the broad picture.

Although the last seventy or eighty years have seen substantial *absolute* improvements in the nation's health, marked class gradients remain in virtually every single indicator of mortality and morbidity. This applies equally to the 'old' diseases of poverty like tuberculosis, which now account for an insignificant fraction of the nation's ill health, and to the 'new' diseases of affluence like cancer and heart

14

disease. There are very few categories of disease where mortality rates for the upper social classes exceed those of the lower and these tend to be somewhat esoteric conditions which are likely to be differentially diagnosed. Between the ages of 16 and 64 a man in social class V is nearly twice as likely to die as his counterpart in social class I. Despite thirty years of the National Health Service, these imbalances have changed little and some commentators have gone so far as to argue that they have increased. Even the sober assessment of the 1971 Registrar-General's Report on Occupational Mobility concluded that, making all due allowances, the position of social class V had apparently deteriorated over the preceding decade. This is particularly disturbing given that we are now into the second generation of the population to be born into a society with a comprehensive health care system largely free at the point of contact. One would expect residual effects from unequal access to care before 1948 largely to have worked themselves out, at least where infant and child mortality is concerned. Yet this has not proved to be the case and, despite an overall improvement, a baby born to social class V parents remains two and a half times more likely to die in the first year of life than his social class I equivalent. A comprehensive and up-to-date account of class inequalities in morbidity and mortality can be found in Hart (1978).

In addition to this concern about inequalities in the incidence of disease and premature death, there has been a continuing discussion of the inequalities in the provision of national health services. In part this is associated with the class composition of localities. Predominantly working-class areas tend to have poorer provision by almost any measure of service standards. But there is also a significant rural/urban continuum. Tom Heller (1978) has shown that some of the most acute service deprivation is in rural areas of the United Kingdom. Taking an overall view, Cooper and Culyer (1972) concluded that regional inequality actually increased between 1962 and 1967. Cooper (1975:64) notes that:

> The health service had successfully dismantled the price barrier but had failed to deal with the others. Inequalities of a geographical nature are unlikely to be any more equitable than those resulting from inequalities in the distribution of purchasing power and clearly there was nothing inherent in the 1946 Act which could have systematically brought equality about.

The situation thirty years after the National Health Service Act remains substantially that characterised by Tudor Hart (1971) in his celebrated Inverse Care Law, that the availability of good medical care tends to vary inversely with the need of the population served. Tudor Hart goes on to observe that the Inverse Care Law is created and maintained by the operation of market forces and their allied ideological superstructures. The degree to which the NHS has failed to modify the law is the measure of the degree to which it has been unable to counter the social forces of a market society. Such redistribution as has been achieved is 'an intervention to correct a fault natural to our form of society and therefore incompletely successful and politically unstable in the absence of more fundamental social change'. As this implies, the distribution of disease and death, on the one hand, and health care services on the other, is a reflection of the society within which health services operate. To adapt Basil Bernstein's (1970) adage, health services cannot change society. The standards of national health which we see today are the outcome of a series of choices about the value which we attach to health and the trade-offs which we make between health and other social or individual goals such as liberty or material well-being (see also Murcott in this volume). These goals, of course, are framed within a particular set of cultural assumptions, allied to a particular balance of material interests. The first task of this paper is to give some account of those assumptions.

Collectivism, Individualism and Social Democracy

Three terms play an important part in this analysis, and it is perhaps as well to begin by explaining what I mean by them. *Individualism* and *Collectivism* are used to describe two contrasting philosophies of welfare provision. In their original Victorian sense, they contrast private initiative and state action. The individualists held a view of society as based on free contracts between individuals very much along the lines of the universal market in classical economics. People were regarded as responsible for their own actions and as ultimately free to exercise whatever choices they liked in disposing of their own lives, provided that they accepted the consequences. The role of the state was limited to providing the conditions in which this market could flourish and acting as a residual arbiter between the exercise of conflicting liberties. Welfare provision was a matter for private philanthropy and should, furthermore, be directed towards the re-establishment of independence and responsibility among its recipients, rather than creating a dependent pauper class. Collectivism tended to be used as a pejorative epithet by individualists against policies of state intervention which seemed to involve the state in restricting the unbridled exercise of economic liberties and in mitigating the burden of individual responsibility. One of the classic debates between the two camps, for example, concerned school meal provision and whether it was right to relieve parents of the obligation to feed their children adequately.

Social democracy is the political philosophy adopted by substantial elements of both the Labour and Conservative parties, although more particularly the former, over the post-war decades. It is essentially a reformist creed based on the principle of the maintenance of a mixed economy, planned on a rational basis of co-operation between private capital and the state but with existing forms of organisation and control and market values and attitudes basically untouched. Public ownership is a managerialist device for maintaining crucial sectors of the economy — power, mining, transport, steel, ship-building, aircraft, docks — where private enterprise has demonstrably failed. The Croslandite emphasis on economic growth to achieve redistribution of wealth is based on a desire to proceed by making everyone richer without making anyone poorer in absolute terms. Without such growth the notion of the redistribution of wealth has no teeth in the sense of bringing about relative change and, indeed, this distribution has altered little since the last war despite fifteen years of Labour government. The imperfections of the market and the adjustments required by social planning are tempered by measures of social reform based on the values of an enlightened bourgeoisie. Comprehensive schooling, in the first instance, was a measure to give 'grammar school' opportunities to all, for example.

In order to understand the development of the NHS since 1948, however, we must understand something of the history of health care in the United Kingdom and the situation which the reform was intended to meet.

Health Services Before 1948

Victorian England was marked by two paradoxical tendencies: on the one hand, this was the heyday of Benthamite individualism as a philosophical rhetoric for the formulation of political action, and, on the other, it saw the widespread development of state collectivism in measures of sanitary reform. Eckstein (1958) suggests three ways of accounting for this paradox. Firstly, he notes that Benthamism was an undogmatic creed which accepted collectivist action if this seemed necessary to optimise *laissez-faire* conditions. Secondly, he contends that the doctrine of self-responsibility was harder to apply to disease which was more clearly a by-product of economic progress. Disease was an indiscriminate threat to all classes and measures to contain it would benefit all. Finally, he argues that public health legislation represented good economy since disease was a major cause of poverty and, therefore, of expense to the Poor Law. While the benefits of sanitary legislation were provided impersonally to society as a whole, the limits of such collectivism were reached at the point where the state might get drawn into the provision of individual medical care, one segment of the society assuming responsibility for another. The controversy over medical treatment in schools offers a good example of this point, paralleling the better-known debate over school meals, in the question of whether the state should relieve parents of certain responsibilities in relation to their children. The eventual acceptance of such a responsibility by the state was to be regarded by, for example, Dicey (1905) as sounding the death knell of Victorian *laissez-faire* individualism.

Private philanthropy and self-help did, however, provide a substantial amount of health care. Private individualism underwrote the voluntary hospitals which provided walk-in health care on an individual basis to the poorest classes. The richer classes were cared for either in their own residences or in private 'nursing homes' (note the choice of phrase). These provisions were complemented among the respectable working classes by private individualist insurance schemes which principally covered general practitioner services. Such schemes were run on a self-help basis by trades unions, co-operatives and friendly societies and covered only those in regular work, able to pay subscriptions, and involved in this sort of co-operative activity. These individualist efforts were complemented by private collectivism. I have shown elsewhere (Dingwall 1974: 77-136, 1977a) how health visiting, for instance, originated in private schemes for district visiting and health and social education on a collective basis, without test of means or need. The consequence of this patchwork of provision, in Eckstein's (1958) view, was that the group most in need of health care reform were the middle classes, socially excluded from self-help insurance, and neither poor enough to qualify for free care nor rich enough to absorb medical bills without concern.

Certain reservations need to be made here. There is a danger of underestimating the degree of self-interest behind both public health legislation and private philanthropy. Legislation was seen to bring direct benefits to the classes which promoted it. These benefits were not peripheral matters like the indiscriminate threat from epidemic disease or Poor Law taxation. They related to matters of central capitalist concern: the quality of the labour force and, hence, the armed services, and the control of the lower classes. Gilbert (1966) shows how the most radical phase of state collectivism under the 1905 Liberal Government, the origins of the welfare state, in his title, was motivated by specific anxieties about military and commercial weakness and social indiscipline. The state assumed direct responsibility for parental tasks, notably in maternal and child welfare, and created agents, like health visitors, to enter and inspect homes with the remit of producing certain changes in family life. These measures may have brought real improvements in the quality of working-class life, but they were only rendered politically feasible by specific class concerns about military failure, international commercial competition and the rise of an indigenous socialist movement. State collectivism was designed to ensure 'The men employed in factories and so on would be fitter as soldiers and the women would be fitter to be mothers of soldiers' (HM Principal Lady Inspector of Factories 1904) and, to borrow Balfour's phrase, to be the social legislation that would act as an antidote to socialist legislation.

Private philanthropy, too, was not prominently altruistic. There was a certain amount of private collectivism for much the same reasons as those outlined above, although there were also socialist and feminist self-help groups which had more radically collectivist goals. But the private individualism which financed the voluntary hospitals was intimately concerned with their role in providing trained and experienced health care personnel for the rich. The great teaching hospitals were in working-class districts, not merely to serve the poor but also to provide suitable clinical material for training and, later, research. The market influence should be obvious. Where else would a teaching hospital be located than in a place where there was a substantial density of sick people? So long as hospital-centred health care retains its pre-eminence, this is precisely the sort of distribution of facilities one would expect to find. Altruism was not, of course, entirely absent. Clearly some of the supporters of the voluntary hospitals were disturbed by the fate of the indigent sick. It is striking, though, in looking at appeals for subscriptions, how these employ a rhetoric of self-interest which, presumably, was expected to be the strongest motivator for potential donors. The historian of the Royal Cornwall Infirmary (Andrews 1975:76-7, 85-8), for example, records how a programme of nurse training on the Nightingale model was financed by soliciting contributions from local notables through an appeal based on the benefits of thus creating a pool of competent women for private nursing duties. The barriers to medical care for the poor were still considerable. One of the most significant was the geographical distribution of services. While the city poor might be reasonably well served, their counterparts in the country and the industrial towns were relatively neglected. The middle-class suburban dweller might have difficulties in getting access to specialist care and be charged over the odds to subsidise the consultants' charitable activities. On the other hand, he would have access to reasonably competent general practitioner services which were sufficiently competitive to keep charges down, to a level indeed where it has been argued that many GPs were seriously underpaid. The poor had to choose between the voluntary hospitals with their attendant inconveniences and unpredictable risk-benefit ratio at the hands of inexperienced or adventurous doctors or the Poor Law hospitals with the associated stigma and relative low level of medical and nursing competence, given the financial pressures to which they were subjected.

The consequences, however, are indisputable. As the work of Eckstein and others makes clear, by 1946, the nation's medical services were thought to be in a deplorable condition. There was a substantial national shortage of beds and equipment and of trained manpower, medical, nursing and paramedical. What facilities there were, were unevenly distributed both geographically and functionally without reference to local need. Most beds were in small, inflexible general hospitals and there was a dearth of provision for both chronic care and complex acute care. This is a predictable consequence of the relatively free market in health care. In competitive situations there is a tendency towards product uniformity, as entrepreneurs compete for shares of the largest market sector. Up to a point it is not rational to provide for minorities, since a small share of the majority market exceeds the size of catering to the whole minority (Lipsey 1966:386-9). Donors, of course, were also more attracted towards small units where their contributions might have a more visible effect or generate some feeling of proprietorship.

Doctors were similarly maldistributed. The availability of private practice concentrated specialists into a few fields in large urban centres. General practice followed suit gravitating towards areas with a congenial clientele and the availability of an autonomous fee for service practice rather than the felt constraints of insurance or contract practice in working-class areas or the social isolation of rural areas.

These difficulties were compounded by the disorganisation of the system. There was no effective co-ordination to promote joint planning and co-operation in specialist service and equipment provision or to prevent wasteful duplication. Administrative boundaries were drawn without reference to provision or need. Moreover, the whole system was impoverished. The public spending cuts of the Depression and the cessation of large-scale building during the War had starved the entire public sector, both hospitals and community, of capital investment. The voluntary sector was in equally desperate straits. Private philanthropy could no longer meet the costs involved and the hospitals were propped up by government payments. The medical profession was similarly impoverished, as were the nurses.

Pressures for Change

Appalling conditions in themselves do not, however, generate change. Their being recognised as appalling depends upon some implicit notion that things might be other than they are, thus providing a standard of comparison. In this case we must recognise the genuine advances that were being made in medicine and surgery. Effective drugs and safe procedures were becoming available and medicine was reaching the point where its intervention was often more successful than not. These benefits, of course, were becoming available through medical research, principally in the voluntary teaching hospitals. The consequences of this for individual charity patients were unpredictable, but the ready availability of human subjects for experimentation undoubtedly contributed to clinical advances. There is a moral trade-off here between extending knowledge to the ultimate benefit of all citizens and the prospects for the predominantly working-class patients who act as guinea-pigs. When Eckstein emphasises that the strongest advocates of change were the voluntary hospitals and the British Medical Association, then this is not merely an indicator of self-interest but also that these are precisely the sectors one would expect to become aware first of the new possibilities of medicine. To implement these generally, new facilities would have to be provided which would demand substantial investment and, given the financial pressures on the services, a degree of co-ordination to achieve a more economically rational form of organisation. In this paper, however, I want to concentrate on the socialist versions of medical reform and their relation to the Labour Party which eventually introduced the relevant legislation.

The plurality of 'versions' is important. In so far as nineteenth-century socialists addressed the question of health at all, it was to regard it as a by-product of capitalism. The provision of free medical services missed the essential point; disease was the outcome of production for profit rather than for use. Under socialism, production would be so ordered as to prevent disease ever arising. This concept of prevention was not the narrow hygienist conception of remedial environmental intervention but, rather, a positive one of producing a society which would, as it were, design out health risks.

The most substantial group of early socialist writings on health is that of the Fabians. They were highly suspicious of the ethics and intellectual standards of the medical profession. This is not without concrete justification. Curative medicine was still in a primitive condition right up to the First World War and in many peripheral areas for a good while later. But the Fabians were genuine radicals; they wanted to reform society, not merely redistribute existing wealth. In this context what are often dismissed as eccentricities such as vegetarianism should be seen rather as part of the new health-promoting life-style which the new society would adopt. The programme set out by the Webbs in *The State and The Doctor* (1910) is a pre-eminently environmental programme where curative and hospital services are residual elements dealing with those circumstances where community provision breaks down. The environmental emphasis also coincided with the Fabian distrust of the working classes. The Webbs argue against free medical treatment, for example, on the ground that it would be abused by the poor. Environmentalism could be elitist social engineering, obliging the poor to live better lives in spite of themselves.

The Labour Party itself had little to say on medical reform, although it supported Lloyd George's health insurance scheme for the benefits it would bring the Trade Unions. By the mid-thirties, however, the Party's position had clearly become one of commitment to free medical services. Its views were more strongly oriented to cure than prevention and there was an active and accepted group of doctors, the Socialist Medical Association, affiliated to the Party.

Eckstein's view is that this is part of a general conversion of the Labour Party from a 'reformative' to a 'redistributive' philosophy. Rather than seeking to reconstruct the social order anew, it accepted the fundamental structure of a non-socialist society and sought to influence the market distribution of goods and services without altering the underlying economic relations and their associated values. There was a preference, for instance, for providing a state education system to allow 'equal' access to education without redistributing wealth, rather than redistributing wealth to allow every parent to buy private education. The provision of state facilities benefited those at the margin, whose means were stretched to finance private services, but did little for those further down whose means limited their ability to profit from this provision. Hence the well-known observation that the middle classes have done best out of the post-war welfare state. In the terminology of this paper, these years saw the shift of the Labour Party from a 'socialist' to a 'social democratic' approach. The nature of this historic compromise and the reasons behind it raise issues which cannot be explored in depth here. Nevertheless, we can note certain features: the concentration on parliamentary power as the means of achieving reform, the basic acceptance of some kind of market economy, the policy of seeking alliance with white-collar and middle-class groups who had a sufficient stake in society to distrust revolution but were not averse to supporting redistributive reforms from which they expected to benefit.

The social democratic programme on health care is a good example of this approach. It aimed at redistributing access to what was now beginning to be genuinely effective curative medicine, particularly to the middle classes whose position was becoming strained by their exclusion from insurance schemes. It gave a lower prominence to environmentalist approaches to public health and the collectivist rhetoric of social engineering which they implied. Instead it took up the market economy theme of bourgeois individualism and adopted individual hygiene as the basis of public health programmes. Finally, it left the prevailing organisation of services and the interests vested in that substantially untouched (see also Davies in this volume). The medical profession was to preserve its autonomy and lack of accountability and retain a position of social privilege. This philosophy was enshrined in the platform of the Socialist Medical Association adopted by the Labour Party in 1934 and still the principal manifesto for its health policy.

It was a platform, however, the basic features of which had already been outlined by others and the acceptance of which was already widespread. In its basic conception of a state-financed and rationally planned health care system substantially free at the point of contact it reflected rather than anticipated a consensus of informed opinion.

The National Health Service

As Titmuss (1958) has observed, the exigencies of war have provoked most of the major advances in the welfare state. The Emergency Medical Scheme brought about the first systematic collection of information about health care provision and revealed the full extent of its acknowledged inadequacy. Evacuation was also a forceful reminder of the living conditions in the large urban areas (Isaacs 1941; Calder 1971).

The conjunction of these experiences with pressure from the medical profession itself and the Beveridge Report's assumption that a 'national service for the prevention and cure of disease and disability' would be provided in post-war Britain jogged the Coalition Government and the Civil Service into discussions about the shape of a reorganised health service. The result was a White Paper in 1944 which substantially defined the terms of debate for the next four years and the shape of the subsequent Acts. The precise details need not concern us here, except to note that the White Paper set out the basis of the tripartite system – hospital, community and GP services – which prevailed until 1974, and, arguably, beyond. In doing so what it proposed was essentially a nationalisation measure, where state finance and state planning would overlay an existing structure of service provision without any mandate for radically altering the nature of that provision. In Eckstein's (1958:3) words, the NHS,

> was not instituted, solely or even primarily, because of the distributive inequities of the old medical system . . . it was intended to correct certain desperately serious faults in the organisation and quality of the British medical services rather than in their class distribution.

While this reorganisation might have redistributive consequences, it was not a principal aim. The loss-making and financially exhausted sectors of the health industry were taken over by the state, leaving the remainder to concentrate on the more profitable activity of supplying goods and services to a nationalised industry.

Implicit in this nationalisation measure was the generalisation of a Victorian model of medical practice to the nation as a whole. It is the failure to reconsider the individualism of that model which underlies the inability of the NHS to remedy structural inequality in health.

Strong and Horobin (1977) note how the professional relationship between doctors and bourgeois patients developed in the nineteenth century as a private contract between individuals unmediated by the state. It was an agreement between individual doctors and individual patients, set against a background of ideas paralleling those of classical economics. The laws of health were conceived to be a set of 'natural' phenomena which were not a matter of human agency and, like the 'natural' laws of classical economics, not a proper subject for state intervention. Individual patients were, like economic man, assumed to be perfectly rational and knowledgeable and to act in such a way as to maximise their self-interest. They *chose* to use the service, deciding when they needed help, whom to consult and whether to follow the proferred advice. Within this contract a doctor's duty lay *only* towards individual patients, with whom he had an exchange of quasi-proprietorial rights; each patient had his 'own' doctor and each doctor, in another sense, owned his patients. Other doctors became involved on licence from the patient's general practitioner. Finally, since medicine was not a matter for outside concern, the doctor/patient relationship was confidential, a private rather than a public matter.

One of the consequences of this form of doctor/patient relationship is, according to Strong and Horobin, an accommodative attitude towards clients. Doctors have legal duties towards patients but few powers to constrain patients' conduct. Such a situation encourages a picture of moral neutrality and bourgeois gentility in the relationship. In pre-NHS England, a practitioner's income depended on the size and affluence of his clientele. It therefore paid not to offend them. Even under the NHS, the GP's income is based on capitation which may be some sanction against giving excessive offence, although given the considerable difficulty of changing doctors it is less effective than it might be. Where a monopoly situation prevails, in rural areas, doctors may be reluctant to give such offence as may lead a patient to deprive himself of care, given the lack of choice, or may make life in an isolated community difficult for themselves. There are strong incentives to avoid moralising and be polite to patients, to their face. Strong and Horobin argue, too, that the rhetoric of citizenship, which surround surrounds the NHS, encourages patients to regard this former bourgeois privilege as a right. Moralising attacks patients' status as citizens in a welfare state.

These arguments are used by Strong and Horobin to examine the consequences of recent proposals, like those in 'Prevention and Health: Everybody's Business' (DHSS 1976a). They argue that the moral neutrality of the doctor/patient relationship would be undercut by a philosophy of holding individuals accountable to the state, via the intermediary of the medical profession, for their predicament. The NHS would apparently be shifted in a more collectivist direction as the state assumed a more direct interest in the moral education of patients and in the control of their everyday conduct. Rather than merely nationalising an individualist model, the NHS would seek to intervene very much more in regulating the lives of prospective patients to ease the burdens on the collectivity as a whole.

This approach I propose to term individual hygienism. It is based on an assumption that preventive health is a matter for individual calculation and action. It finds ironic echoes in the anti-medical self-help movements. Both focus on individual responsibility, what individuals may do to help themselves; the former proposing an extension of state control to regulate individual choices and the latter an extension of individual control as an alternative to medical institutions. Yet, in the long run, both are equally unsatisfactory responses to the strongly conservative forces which uphold the existing patterns of disease and treatment in a capitalist society. The social democratic compromise of providing health care on a collectivist basis, financed by taxation and free at the point of contact, while abdicating collectivist responsibility for the causes of disease, is fundamentally unstable. The costs of health care provision are separated from the gains of disease causation. Individuals are indefinitely free to incur health costs, or to inflict them on others for gain, while the collectivity is presented with an indefinite commitment for treatment costs. The escalating costs of health care are the inevitable consequence of the uneasy compromise of collective provision without collective obligation. Individual hygienism is merely another attempt to prop up this compromise and to avoid the revolutionary implications of collectivist environmentalism as an approach to health services. Ultimately, the only stable counterpart of collectivist health care is collectivist intervention.

Public Costs and Private Gains

Individualism in health care maximises the opportunities for private gain at the public expense. Three sorts of private gain act as the conservative forces which impede health care reform: direct gains from the supply of goods and services to the NHS and from the employment opportunities which the NHS offers and indirect gains from the profitable creation of disease.

Like other nationalised industries, the NHS took over a loss-making sector of private enterprise. It is a feature of social democratic thought that the state only acts as a last resort to the market, where some service or good may be socially desirable and the market is unable to provide it. In general, nationalised industries have been starved of capital investment for decades in the interests of immediate profit. The state is brought into provide that investment and, having done so, to provide a general subsidy to the market sector. In order to reduce market sector costs, nationalised industry prices to that sector tend to beset unrealistically low so that consumers of the goods or services continue not to pay prices which will allow for reinvestment. This continues to be met by the taxpayer at large. The NHS is a classic example in that its price to the market sector is effectively zero. Nationalised industries, however, are also substantial purchasers from the market sector. Indeed, the profitable parts of that sector, on which industries to be nationalised depend, tend to be excluded from nationalisation measures. Mining equipment is still bought in by the National Coal Board, for example. In the present context, three industries are particularly prominent – pharmaceuticals, medical equipment and construction. All of these have a substantial stake in individualism.

Drug treatment is a classically individual therapy. It treats environmentally-generated disease in isolation from its causes. Obviously, there are substantial human benefits in relief from pain, suffering and death. This is not an exercise in medical nihilism. Nevertheless, there are also substantial profits. Robson (1972) notes that the trading profit as a percentage of capital employed was 12.5 per cent for manufacturing industry as a whole and 18 per cent for the pharmaceutical industry. Individual companies were making profits in excess of 40 per cent. Similar arguments apply to the less well-scrutinised equipment industry. Again, profits come from dealing with the consequences rather than the causes of disease. Equipment profits are at their most substantial in high-technology medicine, where tens of thousands of pounds may change hands on a single item of equipment. This high technology demands houseroom, provided by the modern hospital. Hospital treatment is, again, reactive, dealing with people who are already ill and in isolation from their natural environment. Hospital building is a profitable business, as is any form of government construction work. The purse behind it is known to be, for all practical purposes purposes, bottomless and vulnerable to the Concorde effect, where the expenditure of massive sums of money may be used to justify further spending in order not to be seen to have wasted the previous expenditure. The profits on drugs, equipment and construction are as much subsidies to the market sector as underpriced power or underpriced roads. Their scale can be seen in the associated corruption; whether criminal, as in the activities of John Poulson, or merely moral, in the free entertainments from drug companies and equipment manufacturers.

Like any other nationalised industry, the basic forms of capitalist managerialism have remained untouched since 1948 and have, indeed, been reinforced by the 1974 reorganisation. Social democracy represents no challenge to the form of capitalism; it merely creates a state sector, paralleling the market sector, where similar forms of action are harnessed to state purposes. A narrow economism in defining the most rational way of providing existing goods and services continues to be the dominant feature of management thinking. Paradoxically, as several commentators have noted, the increasing entrenchment of managerialist thinking has been matched by the development of health service unionism. The NHS is becoming dominated by a conservative corporatism which sustains the vested interests in individualist health care. Since non-hospital medical services are regarded as residual provisions for those matters in which hospital medicine takes no interest, they tend to be regarded as disposable in managerialist thinking. They find few defenders in either administration or unions. Hospitals have substantial managerial bureaucracies and are easily organised by unions since a large number of workers are brought together in a single location. Extra-hospital services, provided to people in their own homes, isolate workers and give them a sense of autonomy, factors which make them difficult to organise. Hence, health service unions are understandably likely to give priority to resisting hospital employment cuts and, possibly, even to promoting hospitalisation as a form of health care delivery. It seems arguable that curative medicine may be more labour-intensive than environmentalist preventive medicine. Where the latter relies on social engineering to design out health risks, many of the indicated measures seem likely to reduce rather than increase demand for labour; substituting machines for men in hazardous industrial processes, for example. With a value-system which accords priority to paid employment, such a development would obviously be unattractive to workers and one would expect their unions to respond to this.

An emphasis on high-technology, curative hospital medicine is precisely that policy which maximises the opportunities for private gain. It demands high levels of state expenditure as indirect subsidies to the market sector and, at the same time, leaves that market sector free to promote ill health for profit. One of the weaknesses of the social democratic ideology is its assumption that a free market in ideas and knowledge based on intellectual competition and individual choice will produce the desired Utopia of a society which adopts the models of the enlightened latter-day Fabian bourgeoisie in which that ideology is rooted. Health education, as is argued elsewhere in this volume, is an inherently individualistic conception of preventive medicine, designed to compete in this market. In practice, of course, a sort of Gresham's Law operates with the profitable promotion of ill-health driving out unprofitable prevention. It is the manufacturers of tobacco products, alcohol, private motor vehicles and the like who generate the profits which allow them to buy access to sources of mass information and who provide the substantial employment opportunities which enlist union support.

It would be misleading, however, to imply that the community as a whole did not participate in the indirect gains from the promotion of ill health. Apart from obvious benefits like employment opportunities, there are indirect gains in lower private costs. Production involves a trade-off between the risks to workers from production processes and the benefits to the community from those particular modes of production. Replacing a process which causes a given level of death or disability by a safer process might well increase that industry's costs and prices. Disregarding the possibility of undercutting by less scrupulous foreign competitors, the net effect of a safer process may be to make the community as a whole poorer. More resources are consumed in production and fewer of the products can be afforded. Decisions about environmental engineering are decisions about resource allocation. How much consumption are we prepared to forego to reduce levels of mortality and morbidity? If we could wave a wand and abolish smoking overnight, would there be a net social gain as the health costs of smoking were set against the benefits – employment, tax revenue, sponsorship of arts and sports, advertising support for periodicals, etc? Promoting ill health, then, may offer substantial gains for a few; it may equally offer us all, as a community, some benefit even where the community bears the health costs of that process.

Inequality and the NHS

By adopting the prevailing individualism of a market society, which the social democratic compromise of the NHS leaves untouched, the health services become committed to the reproduction rather than the elimination of existing inequalities. Recent debates in the sociology of education have a clear relevance here. In a class society, comprehensive education may create equal opportunities for all; it cannot, of itself, ensure that all are equally able to take advantage of those opportunities. Similarly, comprehensive health care may make treatment equally available to all individuals but it can do nothing to ensure that the need for health care is equalised. Individualist health care responds to need; it does not eliminate it. Economic and social inequality is an inherent feature of a market society, for which social democracy plays a merely cosmetic role. In some ways, indeed, it even enhances disadvantage. The individual hygienist approach of present health education shifts responsibility for sickness even more firmly onto individual sufferers. Rather than being mere victims they are culpable contributors to their own misfortune. Could it not be a logical future extension of this that such people should be, in some sense, punitively dealt with by economic or other sanctions?

If we take a holistic view of disease as a natural stage of man/environment transactions, then we become committed to a more radical programme of social reform than few have yet contemplated. Inequality in health care will not be remedied merely by nationalisation. As we have seen, this simply enshrines bourgeois individualism in a capitalist mode of service organisation. It will not be solved by 'community care' or individual hygienist health education. These merely shift around the burden of ill health without attacking its origins. It will not be solved by some programme of worker control, since the interests of health service employees are not necessarily in accord with a system of health care that would maximise equality. It will not be solved just by more 'self-help' or eccentric 'alternative' care. These are insignificant threats to a conception of health which is so deeply entrenched in the master institutions of our society, even where they do not themselves basically embody individualised conceptions of practice. Most 'alternatives' are as decontextualised as any scientific clinical medicine.

Social inequality is deeply embedded in our way of life. Health inequality is simply one facet of that. If we choose to try to eliminate inequality, then nothing less than a reformulation of our present way of life is called for. Even the programmes of modern Western socialism stop short of this. Measures like the nationalisation of the drug industry would, indeed, even aggravate the present situation, magnifying the bias towards individual curative medicine, a philosophy of looking for a pill to dissolve some socially generated evil rather than attacking the evil itself. What is ultimately called for goes to the very roots of our way of life – the way we design and build our homes and factories, the way we plan land use, the way we use our leisure, the way we organise our agriculture. It would break down the artificial barriers between health, environment, industry and the like, exemplified by present patterns of government organisation. It would demand a new priority of social benefit rather than private gain, a new strategy of collectivist intervention rather than individual *laissez-faire*.

This may be a price we are unwilling to pay. The corollary of collectivist intervention to enhance some individual liberties may be to circumscribe others. A healthier life might also be a much greyer and more uniform existence where ultimately community interests come to predominate over individual interests. By the standards we have known in our lifetime it might also be a poorer society. Restrictions on chemical use in farming in the interest of farmworkers' health might reduce yields and limit the availability of food. Restrictions on food additives and preservatives would reduce storage life and dietary choice. Restrictions on atomic development might reduce the availability of power to run the domestic equipment which substitutes capital for labour and contributes to the emancipation of women. Restrictions on the use of radio-active sources would make it harder to check building safety or limit therapeutic intervention. Restrictions on the anaesthetic gases with their risk to theatre staff would take surgery back to pre-Victorian days. The list can be multiplied indefinitely. Our rates of mortality and morbidity reflect our way of life and without changes in that we cannot expect them to alter (see Miers in this volume).

This is not to say that there may not be societies where health risks cannot be severely circumscribed. It is arguable that, under a special set of historical conditions, both People's China and Tanzania have made particular strides in this direction. The average standard of living of their peoples has advanced dramatically and relatively equally. They have enhanced freedom from disease, though at a price in social uniformity which those of us brought up in a market society would find hard to accept. In societies such as these the sort of individual liberties which we might take for granted are treated as secondary to community or national interests. This may be feasible in a society which has been united by the struggle for independence and has retained the moral force of that campaign. It is not clear that this model has anything practical to offer to us in our present circumstances.

The paternalist social democracies of Northern Europe might offer a more realistic model but even here the strain between collective provision and individual liberties has become apparent under the pressures of economic recession. The moral consensus which underpins a more interventionist state throughout Scandinavia may be more difficult to create in a nation the size of the United Kingdom where citizens do not share in a high standard of living. In dealing with the health problems of immigrant workers, the Scandinavians have had to face the same dilemmas as ourselves. To what degree are they prepared to forego various benefits in the interests of safer production? To what degree are they justified in intervening in people's lives in the interests of some alien moral consensus?

Nevertheless, it is perhaps time to reflect more critically on the rhetorical smokescreen of the egalitarian claims of British social democracy. The NHS is often regarded as the paradigm of social democratic reformism. Its strengths and weaknesses derive from the ideological context in which it was created and developed. The uneasy compromise between collective provision and individual freedoms is a predictable consequence of this ideological confusion. The available remedies, however, are easier to formulate than to implement. On the one hand, we could have a much more thoroughgoing individualisation of health costs so that individuals bore the consequences of ill-health-inflicting actions in a more identifiable fashion. Strong and Horobin's interpretation of the policy embodied in recent DHSS documents points in the direction of a health police role for the NHS but there are alternatives. The most obvious is a return to private initiative in health care. To a casual observer of the American scene, the greater concern for preventive health measures of an individual nature – consuming polyunsaturated fats, taking additional exercise, etc. – whether of proven benefit or not, seems to be related to the substantial individual costs of sickness in a society with limited welfare provision. This concern could be underlined by a prohibition on health insurance schemes which otherwise tend to reduce the individual cost of treatment at the point at which it is sought. The overall aim would be to encourage individuals to optimise their personal trade-off between life style and health, uncomplicated by state or private insurance incentives to reduce the perceived costs of illness. Alongside this would go a fairly strict system of liability to allow individuals whose health had been damaged to recover the costs of their illness from those whose actions or products had caused the damage. Again, one would have to prohibit insurance schemes in order to ensure that the real costs of health-damaging activities were felt directly by their agents.

The limitations on such a scheme are fairly obvious. How can individuals arrange long-term investments to cover themselves against the costs of unavoidable sickness? What about chance congenital abnormalities or diseases whose causation and prevention are obscure? What happens if an illness-producing agent goes bankrupt in the face of claims from sufferers? At the same time, it is a defensible and stable response to the individualist attitudes which constrain the NHS.

The collectivist option is equally problematic. It requires us to concede that the Victorian socialists were right to regard most disease as a by-product of capitalism, a society organised on market principles of self-interest and allied ideological superstructures of private rights and liberties rather than on principles of communal welfare. The demise of capitalism might allow us to achieve substantial reductions in mortality and morbidity with a health care system actively devoted to rooting out the causes of disease. Curative medicine would then be assigned a residual role in dealing with conditions the cause of which is unknown or which slip through the net of collective regulation. Fabian vegetarianism and its reformulation of everyday existence may have serious ideological lessons in pointing to the degree to which we have been deluded by individualist reformism in regarding it as mere eccentricity. After all Shaw was actually climbing the apple tree he fell out of in his nineties and even socialists cannot legislate for happenings like that.

There is, however, no reason to suppose that socialism would necessarily give collective health an overriding priority over collective wealth. There still remains a trade-off between resources allocated to prevention and resources for education, investment, leisure and the like. The point of trade-off might shift if, for example, defence expenditure were substantially reduced but it could still not be avoided. There comes a time when any society has to choose and the price of a healthier society might be one we were unwilling to pay in terms of, by present values, a poorer standard of living and greater regulation of individual lives.

Inequality in health care, then, reflects the choices we as a society make about resource allocation and distribution. The NHS reflects these priorities and cannot, in itself, change them. In attacking the NHS for its 'failure' to redistribute health care or redress class inequality in mortality or morbidity, we are attacking the wrong target. The NHS is as successful or unsuccessful as the social democratic compromise allows it to be. It may not be the best health service in all possible worlds but it seems to be as good as we are likely to get short of far more radical social change than seems presently foreseeable.

Acknowledgements

In order to avoid overloading the text with footnotes and references, I have not been able specifically to cite many of those who have had a substantial personal or intellectual influence on this paper. Apart from those cited and my editorial colleagues, I should, however, record my indebtedness to Mildred Blaxter, Mick Carpenter, Celia Davies, Muir Gray, Malcolm Johnson, Margaret Stacey, Gerry Stimson and Pam Watson. I am particularly grateful to Monroe Berkowitz for his close reading of an earlier draft and his assistance in eliminating some of its confusions and ambiguities. While the use I have made of ideas developed from their work and in our conversations is entirely my own, this present paper would not have been possible without their encouragement and stimulation.

2 HEALTH AS IDEOLOGY

Anne Murcott

Critics have frequently said that the NHS is not a health but an ill health service. Part of their complaint is that it is just a repair service, only concerned when health has broken down. The focus is too narrow, they say; curative services are heavily emphasised at the expense even of services aimed at preventing illness, let alone activities positively promoting health. Although this criticism is familiar, it is also often thought of as recent. While it is, of course, a live concern of the 1970s, it is by no means novel. Such criticism has a history that goes back further than the NHS itself. Curiously, it is a history which tends to get forgotten, so that the criticism has somehow continually to be reinvented. Perhaps the tensions which give rise to it persist, continually recreating the circumstances in which it is found to be relevant. This is, however, beyond the scope of this essay. Here the task is limited to sketching some of the history of such criticism while exploring concomitant difficulties of defining health.

A corollary of this criticism is that health should be considered as something other than merely the opposite of illness. It is more than just the absence of disease. It could be thought that debate about defining health would lead progressively to an ultimate and universal designation. Given sufficient discussion, refinement and reworking, a true definition of health should at last be revealed. But it turns out not to be so. This is an unattainable goal and attempts to achieve it will remain frustrated. For it becomes evident that 'health' is never confined to the realm of biology. Whenever definition is ventured, health is seen to be a state valued not in nature but in society. Nature is not so much indifferent to health, as health holds no meaning in nature. One organism's vitality is another's slow demise; one species' gain is another's loss. Put another way, '(t)he fracture of a septuagenarian's femur has, within the world of nature, no more significance than the snapping of an autumn leaf from its twig'. (Sedgwick quoted in Dingwall 1976:82). Perhaps Sedgwick's comment is a little florid, but it cannot be cruel. Such a valuation is inevitably social and human. What he is referring to is simply the morally oblivious activities that occur in nature regardless of the niceties of culture. Health is essentially valued and known by people.

Certainly those concerned with health, whether as practitioners, teachers or policy makers, do not always offer an explicit definition of health. Both its meaning and its value are taken for granted. Yet, as will be seen, even where implicit, some conception of health is envisaged. Indeed, the kind of health envisaged and the kind of society desired are intricately related. While it may be possible to portray a favourite utopia without reference to a conception of health within it, it seems it is not possible to explore what health means without indicating some preferred form of social arrangements.

The idea that the NHS is only a sickness service is allied to the belief that prevention is better than cure. It becomes clear that its criticism of a narrow, curative orientation rests on a different, more inclusive view of health. But this more expansive view is no less loaded than the narrow one it criticises. It too is a state that is sought after and valued. It too involves preference for certain kinds of organisation of society. It too is born of the social ability to value and to judge. The point is that every commentary on medical states of affairs is similarly a product of social valuation and moral preference. So current criticism of the expansion of the medical sphere of influence, just as much as concern about too narrow a focus in medical practice, of moral and political judgement. Both are morally loaded. It is in this way that health is ideological. Illustrating such a contention is part of the purpose of this essay.

The material is organised chronologically. Choosing a starting date is inevitably somewhat arbitrary, but the nature and focus of this volume makes the decade which saw the inception of the NHS itself a sensible choice. The material is presented in four sections, each corresponding to a decade in the life of the NHS.

The 1940s — Reconstruction

Plans for what would become the NHS were being laid in the 1940s. In the first half of that decade an extraordinary amount of fervent activity was devoted to what became known as Reconstruction. Despite the war, but also because of it, people avidly discussed proposals for the future. In the *Report* which provides an historically logical starting place, Beveridge wrote that a 'revolutionary moment in the world's history is a time for revolutions, not for patching'. (Beveridge 1942:6).

His *Report*, said to be the most widely read and known of any similar publication, was primarily about social insurance. It was also arguably more revealing about the place and significance of health in the proposed welfare state, than was either the 1944 White Paper, which outlines proposals for a national health service, or the 1946 National Health Act itself. While the provision of medical services was to be distinct from social insurance, Beveridge's proposals assume the establishment of comprehensive health and rehabilitation services. Such services were seen as essential to success in social insurance. Accordingly, Beveridge deferred discussion of the administrative details of such services and paid attention instead to the case for his assumption.

He appears to have considered this case as more or less self-evident. He argued that it will be in the state's interest, when high disability benefits are to be paid, to have the smallest possible number of claimants. In one way or another, disease, accident and disability have to be paid for; insurance is costly and so is idleness and lost production. If disability payments are to be universally available, so too must be the medical means to curb these costs.

Although left implicit, Beveridge's vision of health was distinctive; it was also distinctively limited. While health is deemed valuable, he took its value to individuals for granted, concentrating instead on its value to the state. The proposed service was to deal not only with the prevention and cure of disease, but also with disability where it will cover 'rehabilitation and fitting for employment by treatment which will be both medical and post-medical'. (Beveridge 1942:158). In this way he reinforced the point that what is valuable is the maintenance of a healthy and thus productive population.

Beveridge's only concern with this service was that it promoted a fit population in general, and a fit workforce in particular. While he mostly used the words *health* service, rather than *medical* service, and referred to prevention as well as to cure, effectively he did not discriminate. As far as Beveridge was concerned, health and medical designations were virtually synonymous, and prevention no different from cure, *in as much as* the rationale for both was to maintain a healthy citizenry.

Beveridge's conflation of rehabilitation, prevention and cure, was not universally shared. An argument for a vision of health resting on a distinction between precisely these orientations was published in the same year as the *Beveridge Report*. Again in the spirit of Reconstruction, the 'intelligent' reader of 1942, 'without medical training', was promised on its dustjacket a book that could be followed 'without difficulty and . . . with enjoyment'. Arnold Sorsby's *Medicine and Mankind* only obliquely referred to the war. He took a longer view which is part of a tradition that sees medicine as socially important. Sensing the imminence of a new era, Sorsby noted that the growth of medicine had matured, leaving behind what he called a chaos tinged with philanthropy. He foresaw instead that planning and organisation would transform medicine from 'limited individual action into a social function with limitless prospects'. (Sorsby 1942:173). He diagnosed several national ills: persistent poverty, stagnant living standards, a declining birth-rate and general social disorder. Medicine, he reminded his readers, has its roots in human suffering. In trying times it must, more than ever, become a force for social as well as individual ameliora-tion. But in so doing it must doctor itself. For he considered that the ills of contemporary medicine derived from the continuing focus on cure rather than prevention.

> Medicine still looks mainly to healing rather than to avoidance of
> disease; this is a negative view of life dictated by the graveyard.
> (Sorsby 1942:200)

This was a key theme of commentary in the forties. Sometimes it was truncated to a shorthand 'prevention rather than cure'. But it also went further than concern with ill health, i.e. health only when absent, whether cured or prevented. Its essence was a concern to inspire a vision of health, positively promoted and actively sustained.

The 1944 White Paper appeared to endorse this position, roundly putting the case for a new attitude:

> Personal health still tends to be regarded as something to be treated
> when at fault, or perhaps to be prevented from getting at fault, but
> seldom as something to be positively improved and promoted
> and made full and robust. (Ministry of Health 1944:5)

But the document's proposals were artlessly introduced, and belied its own argument. It presented an impressive list of facilities to be provided by the new service; the care of a family doctor, the skills of a consul-tant, laboratory services, treatment in hospital, advice available in specialised clinics, dental and ophthalmic treatment, drugs and surgical appliances, midwifery, home nursing and 'all other services essential to *health*' (my emphasis). Stated like this, these emphasised treatment, cure and repair, rather than prevention and 'health'. Indeed, if health rather than illness figured in the document, it lay more between the lines than its own appeal for a new attitude might have suggested.

The BMA was not impressed. Effectively, it considered that the government had condemned itself out of its own mouth. It too considered that the emphasis of the White Paper was on disease rather than health, and that little was said about preventing illness. Thus provoked, it appointed an 'influential Committee to prepare an authoritative statement' of the 'profession's view on the basic principles of health'. The results of the Committee's deliberations were published as *A Charter for Health*. Prefaced by an appealing photograph of a robust toddler, naked except for her sunhat, it propounded that

[G]ood health is not entirely, or even mainly, a question of medical services. It does not depend so much upon hospitals or clinics or doctors or bottles of medicine or organisation as upon a suitable environment and a proper attitude towards health. (BMA 1946:5)

Yet once stated, the Charter's argument was left undeveloped. Its view of health remained elusive. No more was said beyond identifying its value alongside the desirability of promoting human welfare, national prosperity, happiness, and power. In this sense the Charter too was not really about health at all. It was about *disease*, its insufficient containment, its inequitable distribution in populations. Improvements in housing, levels of income, diet, were all to be promoted as means of preventing *disease*. Achievement of prevention was to be safeguarded by a range of prescriptions for appropriate living. So that in the end, when the Charter was not talking about disease, it was talking about morality and ideology – a blueprint for a good society.

This society would provide a good life in which its members raised their psychologically well-balanced children in a 'house which is also a home'. To this end, the right kind of education for girls was heavily emphasised. Their school subjects, biology and art, chemistry and English, law and history, were all to be 'related to building and maintaining a home and to the nurture of children'. Indeed the main rationale of girls' education was to be home-making; it was to include helping acquire 'good taste in appearance, clothes, furniture, manners and morals, which will be of more value to them in home-making than academic knowledge', In this society a national policy for full employment was considered a prerequisite for the application of a Charter for Health. There were essential factors in occupation considered necessary to the health needs of the individual. One of these was that employment should be neither beyond a person's capacity nor below it. 'Maladjustments of this type are one of the causes of both ill health and delinquency.' (BMA 1946:46-7).

Effectively, the Charter's main emphasis is on an identifiable moral and political philosophy. While the right kind of environment must be developed by private enterprise and by Government policies, ultimately it is the responsibility of the individual to make the best use of it. It is the individual who should strive to achieve a high standard of positive health to enjoy life and reap its full benefits. To this end, people should reconsider their present scale of values, and their attitude towards family life.

[For] the prosperity, happiness and power of a nation are based on the exertions and standards of values of its individual members, and those depend ultimately on the standards of the nation's health. (BMA 1946:92)

In an important sense, there can be no 'neutral' definition of health. There can be nothing intrinsic to a notion of health that necessarily leads to the same moral and political position as the BMA Charter. Rather, that, or any other, position is logically prior and so shapes the view of health proposed. A delineation of health will be formed and informed by whatever moral and political ideology is already espoused.

The point can be illustrated by looking at a contrast found in a pamphlet which, while not dated, must have appeared somewhere between November 1942 and the end of the War. In the same spirit of Reconstruction, it is part of a series the aim of which is to encourage organised discussion of social, economic and political issues arising out of the War. Its author J.N. Morris, then a major in the army's medical corps, considered that 'Everyone seems agreed that Health wants Reconstruction', and that 'the pre-war position must be examined to discover what was wrong 'so that in Reconstruction the mistakes will not be repeated' (Morris n.d.: 1 and 5).

For him, health was supremely social. While acknowledging that physical constitution was inherited, he argued that this matters less than what is done with it. However good and healthy a constitution someone may be born with, life in a poor environment will turn it bad and unhealthy:

We have learned to associate health with an *environment* that satisfied man's needs, ill-health with one that distorts and denies them. Whether our needs are satisfied and how they are satisfied is more and more socially determined; so that if we speak of health and ill-health as *social* functions we are not far from the truth. (Original emphases. Morris n.d.:1)

If the environment is bad, housing poor, conditions of work bad, people poor, then the blame lies somewhere in society; for the quality of the environment is amenable to social manipulation. This view, like that expressed in the BMA's Charter, recognised the importance of environment. Where they differed was that in essence the Charter viewed health as a (biological) phenomenon affected *by* the environment, while Morris in effect viewed health as *constituting* the environment. Consonant with this, Morris' position was collectivist, rather than the BMA's individualist. (See also Dingwall in this volume.) Morris insisted that society largely determines health.

[I] ll-health is not a personal misfortune due often to personal inadequacy, but a social misfortune due more commonly to social mismanagement and social failure. (Morris n.d.:1-2)

Whether ill health be identified as a consequence of the inappropriate attitude of individuals or as a consequence of the failure of some larger social institutions, it does not depend on anything intrinsically to do with the logical categories of disease, illness or health. Either way it emerges from culturally inherited views of the nature of society.

The 1950s – Reconsideration

After the War planning continued and free medical services eventually became available in 1948. The fervour of Reconstruction rapidly died, and a major problem of the NHS emerged. The jokes about a toothless and myopic population stopped being funny, as concern about the cost of the Service mounted. Not only did the matter provoke reconsideration of the nature and management of the Service, it entailed a reconsideration of the vision of health itself. To be sure, the themes of the forties continued; textbooks enshrined the study of the impact on health of the environment, extolled the virtues of 'social medicine' and reminded students of the role of prevention *vis-à-vis* cure (cf. Ross 1952, Brockington 1954). But these remained as incidentals to the major debate.

The issues of this debate can be simply stated. Beveridge, amongst others, argued that because economic barriers to medical care existed, people's health was worse than it need be. Once the barriers were removed, an initial backlog of repair work would be required for those conditions which had been neglected because attention could not be afforded. But after this immediate call on the services was dealt with, people's health, by virtue of the very extension of the new service, could improve. This would happen because medical intervention would be instituted at an early stage of illness, and so avert a greater deterioration in health. Disease was not thereby eradicable, but could be far more effectively contained. This reduction of the reservoir of disease requiring treatment would mean a reduction of the call on the new health service, and thus a reduction of its cost. An ever cheaper health service together with an ever healthier population was promised – the prospect had considerable appeal.

Right from its first full year of life, the NHS cost more than estimated and it continued to do so, under both Labour and Conservative Governments. The tremendous and unpredicted demand for free dentures and spectacles did, however, appear to be finite, and was already levelling off before the imposition of charges designed to curb it. On the other hand, demand for, and the cost of, drugs and other services continued to rise. An Enquiry into costs was officially launched by the appointment in 1953 of the Guillebaud Committee.

The Committee reported that, far from costing more, the NHS was at worst (at constant prices, per head of population) costing the same as in 1949 (Guillebaud 1956). But this conclusion served to refocus attention on Beveridge's vision. Guillebaud warned that any idea that the service would be self-limiting was an illusion. Beveridge's rudimentary cost-benefit analysis failed because the factors he built into it were inadequately conceived. Not only did he appear to have a touching faith in a near total efficacy of medical practice; more significantly, he viewed health as finite.

This view had been attacked earlier in the fifties. Ffrangcon Roberts berated those foolish enough to share Beveridge's views. First, he noted that any success of medical treatment itself created further demand for treatment.

> Every new vista reveals further vistas: the further we travel, the more distant the horizon. (Roberts 1952:55).

Second, he pointed to another never-ending process. As soon as people achieved a higher standard of health, they would expect a still higher standard. Yesterday's improvements would become today's baseline from which to demand additional improvements. All of this was compounded by what Roberts called false distinctions made between health and ill health. In a time of shortages generally, the consequence was to change 'ordinary commodities into medical needs' (Roberts 1952:192). All these factors serve to inflate medical costs.

In this it is evident, incidentally, that Roberts assumed that health was identifiable, and also that medical needs could readily be distinguished from ordinary commodities. His complaint that false distinctions were being made is significant, and foreshadows themes developed more extensively two decades later. He took the view that things medical must be kept in their place; if they were not, then the costs of medical services would inexorably rise.

Ffrangcon Roberts's morality and political philosophy is reminiscent of the BMA Charter of the forties. But where the latter looked forward in hope, Roberts looked forward in foreboding and with warning. While he believed a free and comprehensive health service to be a noble ideal, he regarded it as unattainable under prevailing conditions. What he saw was a challenge to people to exercise restraint and unselfishness. People would only become worthy of the services offered, when they recognised that such services could only be supported by adequate national production. By this, it is not immediately clear whether he meant people to be restrained and unselfish in the call they made on services available, or whether they were to be restrained in eliminating what he referred to as inflationary tendencies of restrictive practices, strikes, lock-outs and go-slow tactics — wich he viewed as limiting the growth of national production. In all likelihood, he would have commended both. Whichever he may have meant, and whatever the merits of his analysis, or the acceptability of his exhortations, it remains inescapable that it was to the realm of the moral and the political that his discussion invariably returned.

Further criticism of too static and finite a view of health appeared right at the end of the decade. Where Ffrangcon Roberts's challenge is perhaps idiosyncratically presented, Dubos's *Mirage of Health* carried the ambivalence of the visionary. His ability to see utopian possibilities allowed by that very token the simultaneous realisation that they remained utopian and thus unattainable. Perfect health was an illusion; mystically he lamented that

> Complete and lasting freedom from disease is but a dream remembered from imaginings of a Garden of Eden designed for the welfare of man . . . (Dubos 1959:11)

He pursued the metaphor of illusion. It was ironic that while modern Americans boast of the scientific management of body and soul, their expectation of life had not increased for several decades, medication was costly, and hospitals could not be built fast enough. But perhaps such boasts were sustained not so much by illusion as by something more serious. So Dubos wondered whether indeed the very supposition of superior health was not itself rapidly becoming a mental aberration.

Is it not a *delusion* to proclaim the present state of health as the best in the history of the world, at a time when increasing numbers of persons in our society depend on drugs and on doctors for meeting the problems of everyday life? (Dubos 1959:29)

Here again are raised questions about what are properly to be counted as health matters. It seems that Dubos too assumed that health problems could be distinguished from everyday problems of living. Somewhere, he implied, something has gone wrong that people seek medical care for non-medical difficulties. Were we not mad to think that we had achieved a superior standard of health when people were behaving in this curious manner? Such questions of propriety, of course, continue to exercise commentators in the seventies.

Predictably Dubos was clear that solving problems of disease was not the same as creating health. At the same time his discussion stressed that thinking about health must take account of a certain fluidity. He adopted a view which identified health — and happiness — as the expression of the manner in which the individual responds and adapts to the challenges met in daily life. This reflected his identification of biological success as a 'measure of fitness, and fitness requires never ending efforts of adaptation to the total environment' (Dubos 1959:32). Given that the environment itself was always changing, so then was the kind of fitness required, so then was the nature of health and the manner of striving for it. Thus we deluded ourselves in fancying that health could ever be achievable. It might be comforting to imagine a life free of stresses and strains in a carefree world but

this will remain an idle dream. Man cannot hope to find another paradise on earth because paradise is a static concept while human life is a dynamic process. (Dubos 1959:221)

The euphoria of Reconstruction had given way in the fifties to reconsideration. Idealism in the previous decade had helped to produce the attractive analysis that the cost of curing would be self-liquidating. The experience of the first few years of the service started to dispel that hope and the euphoria evaporated in the face of Roberts's and Dubos's re-analysis of the problem.

It may be that the work of Dubos, and to a lesser extent Roberts, have been given greater emphasis here than they received at the time. Attractive, even if not established, ideas die hard. Six years after Ffrangcon Roberts published, the Minister of Health was still able to reiterate a variety of Beveridge's views. Speaking in the House of Commons on 30 July 1958, he anticipated an increasing return on investment in health. For by aiming at prevention, and, if possible, elimination of illness '. . . better health will go hand in hand with a diminished cost, and we shall be able successfully to discharge both our social and our economic duty' (quoted in Jewkes and Jewkes 1963:5). Even though his emphasis was on preventing rather than curing illness, the view once again was that health was finite. The discussion was only about better ways of achieving health and presumed beneficial economic consequences; it was not about whether health itself could ever be identified before even starting to devise ways of achieving it. The reconsideration of Beveridge's implicit conceptualisation of health was limited; for the moment, the idea offered by Dubos and Roberts of health as infinitely elastic was overlooked. Reconsideration remained to be pursued.

The 1960s – Reconsideration Pursued, Retrenchment Proposed

The costs of the NHS continued as a major focus of attention into the 1960s. Early in the decade, a pamphlet appeared in which the relationship of the health services to national economic prosperity was again examined. The authors summarised diametrically opposed opinions of this relationship: one that medical expenditure was a *source* of national prosperity, the other that better medical facilities were simply one way in which the community *enjoys* its national prosperity (Jewkes and Jewkes 1963:6). Their pamphlet was devoted to examining the former restatement of the Beveridge principle that increased health service expenditure would result in reduced cost of the service, better national health and improved output at work.

The Jewkeses acknowledged the difficulties of the measurement necessary in determining whether improved output is indeed achieved. For example, the application of scientific research had helped reduce many lethal diseases, but those whose lives had been saved died later on from other causes (Jewkes and Jewkes 1963:vi). They further acknowledged that, while it may be evident that increased expenditure had not resulted in reduced spending on health, it was not possible to show conclusively whether it had or it had not resulted in improved prosperity. An initial outlay had not brought costs down, but there was no evidence that this may not mean that the nation was better off as a consequence. The amount spent, they pointed out, was not the only feature of spending to be considered. They reiterated familiar themes regarding some forms of spending as more likely to 'pay off' than others; preventive and precautionary rather than curative services; capital expenditure directed towards the saving of labour in hospitals; the training of more dentists and doctors and the general encouragement of medical research.

Here they were quite clear in their view of the role of the state. It has a duty to the citizenry to provide those services generally agreed desirable which individuals for one reason or another do not provide for themselves. For, they argued, most forms of spending likely to bring greatest return were precisely those where individual spending, as opposed to government spending, is impracticable.

It is much more difficult for the individual to take steps to provide new hospitals, medical research or general preventive medicine than it is to pay for his own costs as they arise for drugs, doctor's services or hospital treatment. (Jewkes and Jewkes 1963:viii).

The Jewkeses' conclusions effectively coincided with the view of Enoch Powell, who was Minister of Health for more than three years in the early sixties. His characteristically Delphic style of political and economic thinking led him to a version of the view of health earlier propounded by Ffrangcon Roberts and Dubos. He referred to the 'multiplier effect of successful medical treatment'; the longer people survived, the greater the number of people there were to make even further demands for medical care. In addition, the more medical care was provided, the more people wanted it. 'The appetite' he wrote, 'for medical treatment *vient en mangeant*' (original emphasis. Powell 1966:27). Predictably, then, he took the view that health services cannot produce wealth, so much as wealth makes expenditure on health services possible.

The optimism and hope of Beveridge's vision of ever-reducing health service costs was discredited. Enoch Powell described it as a miscalculation of sublime dimensions, and the Jewkeses declared it a mystery that it could have ever been accepted as likely. Retrenchment was in the air; total costs of the NHS were, in the end, as likely to increase as the costs of any other service provided by the government. In July 1962 the Ministry of Health was elevated to Cabinet status, there to compete for resources with Defence, the Home Office and Education.

On the face of it, reconsideration to the point of retrenchment was confined to this aspect, to this attitude to overall funding. Developments in the form of the service continued to receive attention. This was explicitly taken up in 1963 in a Fabian Research pamphlet, pointing out that the NHS was merely the basis for the second stage yet to come. Thus the greatest failure was not in the service, but in the acceptance of it as presently constituted 'as the final edifice instead of merely the foundation and first stage' (Pavitt 1963:2).

Echoing Morris's war-time discussion, Pavitt called for a shift of emphasis from cure to prevention: the aim is 'positive good-health', not just 'the absence of illness' (Pavitt:4). His concerns inevitably led to discussion of the organisation of service provisions. In this he placed major emphasis on what are, often confusingly, called *community* health services, a description supposed to distinguish them from *hospital* services. Here his view coincided with that of Enoch Powell's ministry. The resumption of major *hospital* construction after the 20 year gap because of the war and its aftermath was to be undertaken complementary to the development of *community* care. Patients were to be discharged more quickly from hospital back into the community, and many geriatric and mentally ill patients would not be admitted to hospital at all but remain to be cared for in the community. (The only exception to this trend was maternity care, where domiciliary care was to give way to in-patient deliveries.)

The sixties also saw a series of major negotiations and restructuring of the position of General Practice. Even at that time, these developments in General Practice were seen as significant. (For a full account see Forsyth 1966.) A gloss is provided by George Godber as Chief Medical Officer who considered it an important step forward. He thought it fitting to include commentary on the wider 'medical scene' in his Annual Report on the nation's health (Ministry of Health 1967). He traced the changes in disease patterns and identified the degenerative diseases of heart and lungs as the major contemporary killers. He also noted improvements in knowledge of mental ill health, and in recognition of the contribution made to physical disease by psychological and social factors. For these reasons 'the family doctor of the future is ... going to be much more concerned with the prevention of disease or at least the limitation of disability from disease' (Ministry of Health 1967:201).

The visions of health discussed in the forties are unintentionally revived during these manoeuvres. Setting up group practices, building health centres, and revising NHS contracts, were all supposed to alleviate the isolation, low pay and inferior status suffered by GPs in comparison with hospital doctors. Morale would improve as the realisation grew that general practitioners were indeed specialists, in generalism. Theirs was the specialist knowledge of the range of problems of health, of the details of family background and of the work conditions of each person in their care. The unit of specialty was not to be eyes or lungs, medicine or surgery, children or the elderly; the unit was the whole person. Health was again a matter of the environment and everyday living – not patients but people.

It might seem that the move away from hospital care reflected pleas for concern with health rather than disease, and with prevention rather may often be so); it
towards whole person medicine represented the rescue of a positive view of health from the retrenchment threatened at the beginning of the decade. But such a suggestion fails to take sufficient account of the moral and political contexts in which these moves took place. 'Community care' not only sounds more humane (and may often be so) it may also be cheaper where many of those doing the work are unpaid wives and husbands, relatives and neighbours (see Taylor in this volume).

Endorsement of whole person medicine was as much a consequence as a cause of the changes in the organisation of general practice. Once again, the vision of health pursued is to be seen as the product of the social and political context in which it was generated. The underlying political and economic forces jeopardised a wholehearted commitment to alternative, 'positive' views of health allowing retrenchment to remain on the agenda.

The 1970s – Retrenchment Pursued

The talk was still about costs. By then as ex-Minister of Health, Richard Crossman lectured in 1972 on the need for planning in order to decide how best to allocate scarce resources (Crossman 1972). Three years later, Barbara Castle heading the same Ministry pleaded for closer co-operation with the doctors than she had perhaps achieved herself, in order to get better value for money in the NHS (Castle 1975).

If anything, the talk about costs got noisier. While the conventional wisdom of the 1970s considered the national economic difficulties as temporary, the present effects of restraint were no less severely felt. By the middle of this decade, the Beveridge principle of reducing costs seemed to have been completely reversed. The DHSS cautiously commented that unless some unforeseen and economical method of treatment was developed, 'curative medicine may be increasingly subject to the law of diminishing returns'. (DHSS 1976a:6). 'The more you get, the less you pay' is replaced by 'the more you pay, the less you get'.

An attempt at implementing Crossman's plea for planning appeared in 1976. A consultative document proclaimed itself as a new departure. For the first time, an attempt was made to establish 'rational and systematic' priorities in the recently reorganised health service. Where earlier Secretaries of State had had to swim against the tide in giving greater priority to community rather than hospital care, preventive rather than curative medicine, this document tried hard to turn that tide. It clearly restated the role of community care in helping relieve pressure on hospital and residential services. Even more explicitly it is the *economic* value of prevention that was stressed.

> It is also important to avoid false economies. There should be increasing emphasis on preventive services . . . the health education programme should be preserved, and . . . expenditure on family planning should increase. (DHSS 1976c:2)

The tone may be less melodramatic, perhaps the morality different, but the sentiment is identical to Sorsby's in the early 1940s.

This was the political and economic climate in which David Owen, when still at the DHSS, repeated the complaint with which this essay opened,

> The NHS has for too long been seen only as a 'sickness service', and we have tended to ignore the positive role of promoting good health . . . (Owen 1976:3)

Later in his book he pointed out that health was not something dispensed by doctors. Rather a new attitude should be fostered such that the NHS was not seen as the sole provider of health. Instead, he proposed that each one of us should develop a responsibility for our own health. Thirteen years earlier, the Jewkeses had been a little tentative:

> It may be that the present . . . emphasis upon the more expensive routes to health . . . will weaken as increasing attention is directed to more healthy everyday habits on the part of the individual. It may be that relatively cheap prevention will come to play a more important role . . . (Jewkes and Jewkes 1963:36)

It probably does not matter whether the Jewkeses' remark was an accurate prediction of, or a source of inspiration for, the programme outlined in the other consultative document of 1976 on *Prevention and Health.* This carried sub-titles clearly indicating the view that prevention was 'everybody's business' and referred to both 'public and *personal'* health (my emphasis). Even though it firmly claimed not to be comprehensive, the range of topics covered was wide. It went beyond early detection techniques, vaccination and health education, to include 'some problems of today and tomorrow' such as smoking, excessive eating and drinking, drug use and sexual behaviour. All, according to the document, were 'preventable problems of our time and in relation to all of these the individual must choose for himself' (DHSS 1976a: 38).

David Owen agreed that government alone cannot be held responsible for prevention. He went further, considering it interference for governments to intervene in such areas because of the sensitive issues of individual freedom that are raised. Echoing the BMA Charter of the forties, health is again being seen as an individual rather than a collective matter. Yet Owen also emphasised the part that the Community Health Councils (CHCs) could play. He considered that these representatives of health service consumers should be pioneering the adoption of the programme for prevention, and promulgating the spirit of its thinking. But this highlights a certain ambiguity in this way of thinking. The ambiguity lies in the simultaneous disclaimer of government interference, with government-inspired prompting of bodies instituted by government.

This is not peculiar to what David Owen had to say in the mid seventies. It is a more general feature of the movement towards so-called consumerism in the health services. This dates back at least to the inception of the Patients' Association in the mid-sixties. Whether concerned with the welfare of children in hospital, or campaigning for domiciliary maternity services to be restored or in the CHCs themselves, consumer- and pressure-groups in this field display an ambivalence. In one way, their members react as patients and relatives. They represent lay responses to professionals, complaining of inadequate information in cases of serious illness, of long waiting lists for minor surgery, and on occasion even engage in advocacy on behalf of an aggrieved patient criticising a doctor. In another way, they learn from the professionals — administrators and nurses as much as doctors. For in representing complaints from the public, they frequently meet unyielding professionals. The responses they receive are couched in professional and technical terms. In order to challenge these effectively, consumers' representatives educate themselves accordingly, in the same professional and technical manner. This kind of contradiction is accentuated by leaving them exposed to the possibilities that the very existence of these groups offers the professionals. As consumer groups seek to deal on equal terms with professionals, so professionals are provided with opportunities to mould their thinking and attitudes. David Owen is not alone in seeking to use the CHCs or patients' groups as channels for influencing consumers.

Renewed attention to prevention as better than cure was only part of the debate about the meaning of health in the seventies. The trend of the decade before, which recognised social and psychological elements in the manifestation of physical disease, had become more firmly established. This is underscored in, amongst other things, the incorporation of social science teaching in undergraduate medical education. Whether this innovation does succeed in educating doctors to such recognition is perhaps beside the present point. There are those, however, concerned that it contributes to a tendency more and more often remarked. For, it is argued, it is part of the ever widening of the medical sphere of influence.

More and more areas of everyday life — which have always had consequences for health — are being explicitly highlighted as health and/or medical problems. Already in 1952 Ffrangcon Roberts deplored the failure to distinguish between medical and other commodities as a source of improper financial burden. For Dubos in 1959 it was crass to be confusing day-to-day difficulties with indications of ill health. Again in the mid-seventies there are those who raised the alarm at the increasing medicalisation of society.

In Britain, Wilson (1975) complained of concern with disease when we should be thinking about health. Worse, our very society is unhealthy, despite claims to have achieved a civilised level of health. Rather, he says ours is a 'sanitated' society; not only is our view of health limited to concern with eradication of disease, we are also guilty of trying to sweep up, away, and out of sight problems of mental subnormality or old age that cannot be solved or cured. Worst of all, we try and hide death. His vision of health is extensive, so much so that he collects, as a summary at the end, the forty or so different descriptions of health that appear in his book. His ideas of health incorporate ideas of goodness, of humanness and personal and social development. Health necessitates suffering, and the acceptance of death is essential to health. At the same time, for Wilson, talking of health means talking of his idea of the good society, just as it meant for the authors of the BMA Charter of theirs.

At about the same time in the United States, Ivan Illich (1976) made the same complaint. Society's health is threatened by the very activities of doctors. Medicalisation of living has reached unhealthily dangerous proportions. Our very culture has become imbued with a medicalised arrogance that leads us falsely to believe in the conquest of disease, pain and death. For Illich as for Wilson, this involves devastating risks because it means the extinction of what is quintessentially human. It is human to suffer; we know we are alive if we are aware of the inevitability of death. If we lose these experiences, he says, then we can no longer remain healthy.

Amongst other things, both these authors demonstrate the fluidity, the elusiveness and the malleability of notions of health. For them health consciously connotes far more than 'merely' the biological. They ally it to peace of mind and personal fulfilment. Indeed they stretch their metaphors so far that effectively their designations of health actually become descriptions of their desired society. Incidentally they contain the ambiguity and ambivalence already noted, to the point of full-blown contradiction. On the one hand Illich, Wilson and others are agitated at the prospect of an increasingly medicalised society. They warn that a 'sanitated' society may be a bad society. They are perturbed as doctors venture more and more beyond boundaries which were once said to mark the medical from the non-medical. On the other hand it is recognised that there will continue to be a sort of 'residual' curative function for doctors. So Illich, for example, wants to see restored to the doctors the benign, caring character of the old 'liberal' professions. At the same time, then, Illich, Wilson and others urge doctors to halt the dehumanisation of medical practice and treat their patients as people not cases. They want the 'whole' person to be taken into account; Nicky Smith is not just another case of tonsilitis and nor is Toby Jones just the broken arm. They want some recognition that matters of health and illness are not reducible to the technology of seeking to eradicate disease and abolish pain. Indeed they advocate their visions of health precisely because they go beyond 'mere' physical manifestation. They want it recognised that, as well as the biological, the environmental, social and indeed spiritual are also involved.

Many people have found that what both Illich and Wilson have to say is immensely powerful and very attractive. Illich's message in particular has enjoyed international attention. Not only can it lend support to criticisms of over-professionalised and over-bureaucratised health — and welfare — provision but can also go well beyond. It fits in with people's worries that society has become too impersonal. It allows them to hope for an improved way of life where one person cares for another. In short, it accords with romantic yearnings for the supposedly lost community. Although the ideas of health of Wilson and Illich may contrast with those of Pavitt, Powell or the Jewkeses, and although their images of health may be alternative to those of the BMA Charter of Beveridge himself, they all have one significant feature in common. They are all valuations, all utopian and as such they are all ideological.

This essay has sought, then, to reveal health as valued, health as desired, health as ideal. A sketch of the first four decades of the NHS traces corollaries of health as ideology. In recognising this, perhaps, future discussions of health will be informed by those of the past. Not only may the lesson finally be learned that the search for a 'pure' definition of health is fruitless, and that excursion into morality, economics and politics is inevitable. Perhaps it will also be learned that history need not be left to have to repeat itself. If people do not want a 'sickness' service, then they need to develop an awareness of whichever visions of health lie implicit in their proposals for health and welfare provision. If people want to develop practicable and fair medical services they need to understand the trickiness of an infinite demand. If they are alarmed at the potential of medicalised society, people must also consider the consequences of continually extending the limits of defining health. Whatever direction discussions of health and developments of medical services take in the next four decades, perhaps they will benefit by the lessons and experiences of the last four, recognising that whichever expression is given to it, 'health' remains as ideology.

Acknowledgements

I am very grateful in the preparation of this paper to my co-editors for their criticisms and comments, to David Held for generously giving his time to advise at the rewriting stage and, in particular, to Bill Hudson for his continuing help, sensible suggestions and wise observations.

3 HOSPITAL-CENTRED HEALTH CARE: POLICIES AND POLITICS IN THE NHS

Celia Davies

Introduction

For those steeped in a tradition of organisational analysis, hospital-centred health care is likely quite simply to connote a bias in the locus of delivery of health care towards the large-scale, usually general, hospital. As such, it will encounter problems common to all large-scale organisations engaged in people-processing: dehumanised treatment, rigid hierarchical staff regulations, inflexibilities, failures of communication, goal displacement and so on. There is, however, a broader interpretation of modern hospital-centred health care which associates it with any or all of the following: a curative rather than a preventive orientation, an individualistic, one-to-one service bias rather than an environmental or population change one, a technological approach and a devaluing of personal skills, a focus on acute and episodic rather than chronic illness, specialised and fragmented treatment rather than holistic care, an urban rather than a rural concentration (Navarro 1976; Draper 1976; Illsley 1976).

Taken together, these biases have been shown to be strikingly inappropriate in Third World settings and their applicability has increasingly been called into question in advanced industrial societies (Illich 1975; Powles 1972; McKeown 1976). Critics draw attention to the underlying model of what medicine is and can do, and see the source of difficulty not in organisational dynamics but in the 'clinical mentality' of the medical profession (Freidson 1970) and/or in the economic and political forces of the societies in which such arrangements have arisen. From such points of view real alternatives to hospital-centred health care are difficult if not impossible to implement without far-reaching social, political and economic changes. The bias connoted by hospital-centred health care is not simply a bias in the locale of delivery of health care, but a bias in the very definition of what constitutes health care. And if this much is allowed, then paradoxically we may have hospital-centred health care and a decline in the actual use of hospitals. Hospital-centredness from this standpoint is not a straightforward variable to measure. It refers to a *type*, not a locale, of care and, as is clear from the brief list above, that type of care itself has a number of dimensions which, though interwoven, demand separate treatment. Much current health policy in Britain is concerned with an attempt to shift resources out of the hospital towards 'community care'. I shall demonstrate below that this plan starts from a position where care is very much focused on the hospital and is meeting with difficulty. I shall go on to argue that the difficulties can be more clearly understood if we see hospital-centredness not just as a locale of delivery, but as a mode of practice deriving from the historically interrelated logics of action of interested parties and beyond which it is difficult for those interested parties to see. This paper then is offered as an effort to explore the dynamic of hospital-centred health care.

The first section of the paper consists of a brief presentation of material indicating the key position of the hospital itself as a centre of health care since the inception of the National Health Service in Britain in 1948. It demonstrates the considerable and continued importance of hospitals as a focus of care. Such a pattern, I claim, was not the explicit intention of health policy. It grew instead from the social relations and social problems of an earlier era. If we are prepared to interpret the term broadly, then 'politics' rather than 'policy' shaped hospital-centred health care. In recent years direct policy making has played more of a part, but it is still a limited part. This is examined in later sections. Hospital-centredness, I shall argue, is a phenomenon which rarely receives overt discussion, and indeed is hardly likely to do so, given the hospital hegemony over training of health workers of all kinds. Paradoxically, the 'community care' now so strongly advocated is hospital-centred again, though in a somewhat different and perhaps even less attractive guise.

Hospital-Centredness, Resources and Resource Use

Commentators both inside and outside the NHS have recognised its hospital-centred character. In a lecture early in 1977, the Secretary of State for social services, for example, referred explicitly to budgetary allocations, pointing out that over the past five years the proportion of total current budget devoted to hospitals had increased from 60 to almost 65 per cent (Ennals 1977). Academics have also produced data on financing, manpower and resource use to underline a hospital bias and to argue for some reallocation (Cooper 1975).

By financial criteria, we find that since the outset of the NHS hospital expenditure has indeed been the largest single item of cost in health and welfare services. The sum total of provision outside the hospital has never reached 50 per cent of the budget and the figure for

Table 3.1: UK NHS Expenditure — Proportion Spent on Each Service[a]

	Percentage												
	1951	1953	1955	1957	1959	1961	1963	1965	1967	1969	1971	1973	1975
Hospital services	55.7	55.5	57.2	56.8	57.1	57.0	60.1	60.4	59.9	63.1	65.3	66.2	65.8
General medical services	9.5	10.8	10.2	9.7	9.2	9.6	8.3	7.8	7.9	8.0	8.1	7.4	6.1
Pharmaceutical services	9.7	9.5	9.5	9.7	10.2	9.8	10.1	11.1	10.6	10.4	9.8	9.4	8.4
Dental services	7.8	5.5	6.3	6.4	6.5	6.2	5.7	5.1	5.0	4.9	4.9	4.4	4.0
Ophthalmic services	2.8	2.2	2.5	2.2	2.1	1.8	1.6	1.6	1.5	1.5	1.3	1.1	1.3
Local Health services	8.5	8.8	8.9	8.8	9.1	9.3	10.0	10.3	10.4	7.8	7.0	6.9	—
Other[b]	6.0	7.7	5.4	6.4	5.8	6.3	4.2	3.7	4.7	4.3	3.6	4.6	14.4
Total	100.0	100.0	100.0	100.0	100.0	100.0	100.0	100.0	100.0	100.0	100.0	100.0	100.0

Notes: [a]The definition of the NHS was changed in 1969 and certain local authority health services were transferred to the social services sector. Reorganisation in 1974 meant the transfer of local health services to Regional Health Authorities ('hospital' and 'other' headings). It should be noted that between 1969 and 1974 LASS expenditure increased by almost 70% in real terms, compared with an increase of under 20% for health services (OHE 1977).

[b]Includes grants, central administration and items such as laboratory, vaccine and research costs not falling within any one service's finance.

Source: Office of Health Economics, Compendium of Health Service Statistics 1977; compiled from Ministry of Health Reports, Annual Abstracts of Statistics and National Income and Expenditure Statistics for various years.

hospitals has consistently been above this. The proportion of expenditure on general practitioner services and other executive council provision has in fact exhibited a downward trend, while the welfare/social service provisions have increased their share (see Table 3.1). As far as capital expenditure is concerned, hospitals at first sight appear to have done less well. Even now, current expenditure constitutes as much as 80 per cent of the total hospital allocation, and in the early years in particular, monies for capital building were not forthcoming. This presented especial difficulties since the NHS inherited much old and outdated hospital building. There was not a single new hospital in the first 13 years of NHS operations. But when capital was available it went to hospitals rather than to other sectors. It continues to do so, as the latest available figures show (DHSS 1976d).

Table 3.2: Growth Trends in Selected Occupations in the Health Service, Hospital and Community[a]

	England & Wales			England		
	1964	1969	% change p.a.	1971	1975	% change p.a.
Hospital staffs						
Medical	18,346	22,001	3.7	22,548	26,922	4.5
Nursing	199,444	230,716	3.0	232,636	280,701	4.8
Midwifery	12,921	15,173	3.3	13,732	15,358	2.8
Physiotherapy	4,009	4,478	2.2	4,424	4,462	0.2
Occupational therapy	1,207	1,564	5.3	1,641	1,809	2.5
Community staffs						
GPs	21,889	21,505	-0.4	20,597	21,752	1.4
Home nurses	8,182	9,304	2.6	9,069	11,665	6.5
Health visitors[b]	5,071	5,565	1.9	6,747	7,423	2.0
Midwives	6,461	5,767	-2.2	5,051	3,220	-10.6
Physiotherapy				247	580	27.0
Occupational therapy				73	135	17.0
Social services staffs						
Social workers	n.a.	n.a.		10,346	16,523	12.4
Home helps	29,005	32,625	2.4	32,550	44,175	7.9
Workers in res. homes for elderly and phys. handicapped	31,970	36,526	2.7	37,684	48,456	6.5
Total PSS staff	n.a.	n.a.		122,600	179,070	9.9

Notes: [a]Figures are whole time equivalents with exception of GPs. They also include trainees with the exception of health visitors 1964 and 1969.
[b]School attached HVs not included.
Sources: Digest of Health Statistics for England and Wales, Health and Personal Social Services Statistics, various editions.

It is conceivable, of course, that the consumption of finance by the hospitals sector could be offset by a concentration of labour power in health outside the hospitals. While it is difficult to produce comparable series of manpower data, available figures suggest this is not the case. Table 3.2 shows that as far as medical staff are concerned it was hospital medical staff who experienced a growth in the 1960s, and a sustained, and somewhat accelerated, growth again in the early 1970s. General Practitioner numbers actually declined in the late sixties and grew only slowly in the early seventies. Local Authority medical staff are not shown, but we are dealing with small numbers here, still less than 2,000 whole-time equivalent staff at the time of writing. If we look at nursing, the community sector (health visitors and home nurses) kept pace in its growth with the hospital sector. However, this expansion was concentrated on home nurses, delivering clinical care, while health visiting continued its existing growth curve and the number of trainees actually fell back from its 1973 peak. The trend to hospital deliveries is witnessed in the growing numbers of hospital-based midwives. Two groups of paramedicals which have some community base are physio- and occupational therapists. Despite their high growth rates, numbers of community workers in these occupations remain negligible. Social service workers have seen the most rapid growth trends of any substantial group of staff.

Table 3.3: Proportion of Total Staff Employed in Hospital Settings, Selected Occupations in the Health Service

	1971	England (WTE) 1975
Medical[a]	45.5%	52.5%
Nursing[b]	90.8%	90.9%
Midwifery	73.1%	82.7%
Physiotherapy	94.7%	88.5%
Occupational Therapy	95.7%	76.1%

Notes: [a]Medical staff include all community health doctors.
[b]Nursing staff include health visitors.
Source: Calculated from Health and Personal Social Services Statistics 1977.

Further perspective on these figures is yielded by a simple calculation of percentages of health staff in the two settings (see Table 3.3). Nursing is overwhelmingly located in hospitals, medicine is increasing in a hospital location. Other groups of staff are concentrated in hospitals too. This is true, of course, for many professional and technical service occupations, for administrative staffs and for ancillary workers, although, viewed in this way, some slight trends towards a community base for paramedical therapists emerge.

If we turn to the statistics of use of health services the nature of hospital-centred care is further clarified. Selected information on hospital use is presented in Table 3.4. While the total of beds in use has decreased, the usage of hospitals has increased. Added resources and technological changes are clearly factors contributing to a more intensive use of facilities. Thus, between 1959 and 1969, throughput (discharges and deaths) increased by almost a third, outpatient attendances increased by 15 per cent and use of accident and emergency facilities by a similar proportion. Day cases first appear in the statistics in 1972 and by 1975 numbered some 422,000. Turning to the more detailed composition of this work, it is accounted for largely by the clinical (acute) specialties. Over the total period under consideration, 1959-75, these specialties retained a steady hold on total outpatient attendances at around 95 per cent, they accounted for around 92 per cent of all discharges and deaths, and at 38-39 per cent of the total, retained their hold over the total occupied beds. These are important points to bear in mind when examining the recent trends. The 1970s have seen slower growth of services, and a decline in use of several facilities. As the Table shows, 'priority' groups such as geriatrics and mental handicap are now growing areas of work, but starting as they do with so few of the total facilities, the overall distribution is not much affected.

A detailed consideration of hospital-centredness in use-data would clearly entail consideration of a wide range of health-related activities outside the hospital, and a fair amount of such material is available (see DHSS 1976b) but the broad pattern of health care since the inception of the NHS is already reasonably clear. Financial resources and manpower have been concentrated in hospitals. Direct provision of medical and related services in the community has grown but has not achieved a greater share of all resources. Some health-related activities, currently reported as personal social services, have grown rapidly of late. Within the hospital-based provision, it is the acute services which have captured the bulk of the resources. Why has this occurred? Consideration of formal policy decisions alone does not prove very illuminating. I have chosen instead to analyse the development of health care with reference to different interests in and usage of hospitals and to start much further back.

Table 3.4: Hospital-Centredness — Trends in Use of Facilities (Selected Indicators)

England '000s.

	1959	1969	1959-69 % inc.	1971	1975	1971-75 % inc.
All specialties						
Total outpatient attendances	27,768	31,801	15	33,129	30,947	– 7
Total A & E attendances	11,582	13,535	17	13,130	12,792	– 3
Average beds occupied daily	389	359	– 8	347	313	–10
Day cases	–	–	–	–	422	–
Discharges and deaths	3,783	4,968	31	5,171	4,976	– 4
Mainly 'clinical' specialties[a]						
Total O/P attendance	26,609	30,191	14	31,407	29,186	– 7
Average beds occupied daily	149	140	–6	136	124	– 9
Day cases	–	–	–	–	395	–
Discharges and deaths	3,514	4,612	31	4,803	4,580	– 5
Geriatric and young disabled						
Total O/P attendance	51	124	+143	149	195	+31
Average beds occupied daily	51	53	+ 4	54	52	– 4
Day cases	–	–	–	–	1	–
Discharges and deaths	131	166	+ 27	173	200	+16
Mental handicap						
Total O/P attendance[b]	–	7	–	12	19	+58
Average beds occupied daily	54	44	+ 2	54	50	– 7
Day cases	–	–	–	–	–	–
Discharges and deaths	6	12	+100	15	17	+139

Note: [a]Excludes all psychiatric cases, geriatric cases and young disabled.
       [b]Excludes all accident and emergency work.
Source: Health and Personal Social Services Statistics 1976.

Hospitals – Nineteenth-Century Concerns

In the nineteenth century it was largely the sphere of public health which generated activity by central governments. Action was hesitant and uncertain; measures were taken cautiously; decisions, once taken, were sometimes reversed. Yet infectious disease and death in the new urban areas pressed itself upon the consciences of many. A sanitary reform movement agitated for changes and gained support from diverse quarters. A Central Board of Health had been temporarily established as early as 1831 to take emergency measures to combat the spread of cholera and Clauses Acts had enabled local action on matters such as gas and water undertakings, provision of cemeteries, regulations on food adulteration, on certain buildings, sewers, refuse disposal, etc. By the end of the century sanitary authorities had been drawn up with boundaries coterminous with the new local authorities. Responsibilities were extending from environmental health regulation to the provision of certain personal health services and also to the provision of hospitals.

But it would be a mistake to think that responsibility for health was a concept which slowly expanded in its scope. In the same way the public health measures arose from changing economic circumstances and were hotly debated in terms of ideas of collective responsibility and the proper role of governments (see Dingwall in this volume); questions about personal health services to individuals, in the home or in the hospital, arose and were discussed within a specifically nineteenth-century economic and political framework. We cannot hope to understand the evolving structure and functions of the hospital without some knowledge of the social relations of the time. One key factor here was the emergence of a more organised and more unified medical profession. Another was the changing social composition of the population and, thus, the changing set of ideas about responsibility for the lower orders and about the threat to social order and economic advance that such classes constituted. We shall see below how these factors came to shape both the extent and the character of hospital provision. Furthermore, hospitals were a local affair; for a long time they reflected the pushes and pulls of local politics and local interests. When central government did intervene it did so by laying powers on local agencies. This too had implications for the nature of services provided.

What then, were the interests of different groups in hospitals? Let us start with the rich, for as far as the rich were concerned, the hospital was at no time in the nineteenth century the preferred locale for their own health care. The sick rich preferred to consult and indeed largely to control a doctor of their own choice (Waddington 1973) and if necessary to hire a nurse for work in the home. It was not until the twentieth century and its advances in medical knowledge that the rich and the newly emerged middle classes made felt their demands for hospital beds (Abel-Smith 1964; Woodward 1974). The sick poor also had recourse to medical practitioners. These were largely the apothecaries and chemists, and later to some extent also the new general practitioners and the Poor Law district medical officers. But, in addition, the poor were to be found in institutional settings. These were of two sorts, the voluntary hospitals and the Poor Law institutions. The voluntary hospitals of the early part of the century were largely the result of lay philanthropic effort. Their inmates were not always infirm, but they were selected by subscribers to the hospital and were subject to a detailed and meticulous regulation of their behaviour such as to produce more uplifted and upright citizens. The ideas of donors rather than the practices of doctors dictated the case mix. The doctors, indeed, were visitors to these hospitals, their main interests lying with private patients outside. As far as the Poor Law hospitals were concerned, inmates too were very varied. The amendments to the poor law in the 1830s meant the possibility of home care or of institutional provision. The balance of interests, at least at first, however, served to institutionalise the sick poor in a mixed workhouse (Abel-Smith 1964; Hodgkinson 1967).

Both kinds of hospital were transformed as the century progressed. The voluntary hospitals grew in numbers under the ready prompting of doctors. Foucault's (1973) research has shown some of the links between the development of clinical knowledge and the concentration of patients for observation in the hospital ward. Waddington (1973) has developed important points about the availability of the powerless poor in the hospitals in Paris as a resource for the doctors in developing their diagnostic and classificatory skills. By the mid-century in Britain, it was becoming increasingly recognised that this new knowledge could be conveniently pursued in hospitals and that a hospital post and the experience it brought could be an asset in building a private practice. Holding a hospital appointment gave the doctor an acquaintance with the hospital trustees which was also a basis for extending private practice. Added to this, was an income from teaching medical students which could be considerable. For these reasons, the growth of voluntary hospitals, teaching hospitals and specialist hospitals was in the interests of the doctors, and, furthermore, filling hospitals with patients helped in the appeal for funds. Abel-Smith (1964:16), from whose account I have freely drawn material, has this to say:

> The growth of the hospital 'movement' was made possible by the
> money given by the public; but the major impetus in channelling
> charitable bequests and donations in this direction came increasingly
> from doctors. They wanted hospitals for teaching and research.

Public hospitals followed a different dynamic of growth, but one
which by 1900 was similarly generating expansion. Provision here had
much less to do with pressures from the development of the medical
profession and much more to do with efforts to keep down the burden
of the rates and to minimise public provision for the poor. Such a goal
was thought to be accomplished by offering the indigent the workhouse, and by making that institution so unattractive as to deter
malingerers. In the terminology of the time the goal was 'less eligibility'
and the means 'indoor relief' rather than 'outdoor relief'. The sick were
caught up in this, and the mixed workhouse was a result. Later, a
number of factors including the filling of the workhouses, criticism of
their conditions and the problem of accommodating the infectious sick
were among the factors contributing to change. The building of separate
hospitals which occurred in the latter part of the century was tied
closely with goals of restoring 'discipline' among the able-bodied poor
and economising by reducing outdoor relief very much further. Abel-
Smith again has a succinct comment, that 'the prevention of abuse was
thought more important than the prevention of the spread of disease'
(Abel-Smith 1964:87). As an employee of the Poor Law Guardians, the
Medical Officer was in a weak position to influence matters, as compared with the growing strength of the hospital consultant with means
independent of the hospital.

How far then, was the hospital the locale of health care in the last
century? The answer is for the rich not at all and for the poor very
much. The reasons for this have very little to do with any central policy
about health as such; they have a great deal to do with two processes:
one the development of medicine and medical specialties, the other
the problem of collective responsibility for the poor. Both processes were operating at a local level to shape the nature of hospitals
and the experiences of patients in them.

The Early Twentieth Century – from Politics to Policy?

To speak of 'the rich' and 'the poor' is at best a shorthand; as we move
towards the twentieth century the need to incorporate 'middling strata'

into the analysis becomes increasingly insistent. Where did these fit? Were they subject to the degradation of (normal) lower-class patient-hood in the hospital, or were they able to employ practitioners to visit them and nurses to tend to them on their own terms in their own homes?

The pattern of health care which had emerged by around the turn of the century was sharply class differentiated. The rich engaged the honorary hospital consultant and paid him a fee. They benefited from his experience in voluntary hospitals where he gave free treatment to the poor. The poor benefited as they could from the provision and from poor law facilities. Health care was largely hospital centred for them. A new group of general practice doctors, however, was gaining a more coherent identity. With a small fee payment or insurance system they gained a living by catering for the relatively affluent. But theirs was a precarious living. They complained bitterly of 'hospital abuse' – the practice by consultants of seeing cases which were interesting but not always strictly indigent in the outpatient facility of the hospital. They chafed at the control that employment by friendly societies or trade union groups meant over their living and practice. Things were to become more complex as both rich and less rich began to see the advantage of hospital care given its medical advances and facilities. This was especially the case with surgery which could no longer be reproduced with ease at home. Again, this was something that threatened the livelihood of the practitioners, unless a strict division could be drawn between hospital work and general practice (Waddington 1977). Matters were soon to be complicated still further with local authorities adding personal health responsibilities to their public health concerns. Dingwall (in this volume) has made reference particularly to the measures of the Liberal Government of 1905 with its interests in maternal and child welfare and health visiting. The practitioners were thus threatened from all sides; though distinct in name, at this time, they had no distinct area of work expertise. Concepts of primary and secondary care came later as McKeown (1971) has shown. In such a context the 1911 National Health Insurance Act was particularly important in shaping the pattern of care. It introduced a limited but nationwide and state-financed service for primary medical care based on insurance principles. Coverage extended to GP services, drugs and medicines and provided a very small cash payment during illness. Certain additional benefits were possible, including hospital care, but they were only available under highly restrictive conditions. Wage earners alone were eligible and the income limit was £160; the unemployed were excluded, so were women and children and any middle-class membership.

From the point of view of hospital-centred health care what did this mean? First, the scope was very narrow; economically the most disadvantaged groups remained with recourse to the hospital as their only option, and the problem of the middle-income groups was not solved. Second, the services were limited. Local authorities, already taking an interest in preventive and inspectional health facilities, expanded into some personal health care too. After 1911, midwifery, home nursing and an extended Medical Officer of Health Department grew in many local authorities, and in 1921 additional powers were granted to provide aftercare for TB cases. Thirdly, the hospital was affected. The voluntary hospitals were able to be more selective than hitherto; they could return trivial cases among insured patients to panel doctors. Though they continued to provide a primary care service to groups not covered by the Act and increasingly became concerned with pay beds and prepayment schemes for the middle classes, 1911 nevertheless was an important step towards the pattern of referral from generalist to specialist which we know today. As for the public hospitals, they grew less rapidly than the voluntary ones in the decade after 1911, and the growth was mainly in those areas of less concern to the voluntary hospitals, namely fever cases, maternity and TB.

These trends, especially those in the voluntary hospitals, are important pointers to hospital-centred health care as we know it today. Under pressure from the doctors, the voluntary hospitals had already begun to be selective, focusing on 'interesting', i.e. acutely ill patients; and this trend away from catering for a social category of patients, the initial intention of the founders, towards catering for specific diseases was accelerated by the legislation. Some hospitals in the Poor Law system were able to follow suit, concentrating on interesting, acute cases and offering possibilities for student training, and for a visiting medical staff (Abel-Smith 1964:354). This meant that future practitioners as well as future specialists were seeing a narrower range of illnesses. Their ideas about good practice and about worthwhile areas of research would inevitably be shaped by this. The 1911 Act might appear at first sight to stem the shift towards hospital-centred health care but in practice it contributed to giving that care its modern character, and moulding the vested interests which were to take part in the shaping of a health service. Furthermore, personal health services outside the hospital were in rather a mess. Not only were they split between the general practitioner and the local authority for some categories of patients, but the local authority was also engaged in some preventive health services as well as public health measures (individual screening in schools for example).

The 1911 Act, as the comments above imply, by no means resolved the question of the availability of health care provision. In particular, it did nothing to stem the rising demand for hospital care, medical advances having made hospitals more attractive than formerly, and the growing wish on the part of the hospital doctors themselves to expand their facilities and competencies. The voluntary hospitals in fact experienced increasing difficulty in trying to cope with their growing popularity. Having developed as a result of private beneficence their distribution and quality were uneven and competition rather than co-operation was the norm. Having operated on the basis of charity patients and unpaid doctors, their position was anomalous. Whether hospitals could survive without some form of control or local government aid was in doubt. In 1921 a bill to create municipal hospitals was lost; but the new Ministry of Health set up an enquiry into the hospitals and a grant was made and a commission set up. Matters were not settled however. Under the 1929 Local Government Act, the local authorities were enabled to take sick care out of the Poor Law and to take over all non-voluntary hospitals. Conceivably they could have done this, and could have produced a system of hospital care which integrated chronic and acute care. For various reasons they did not do so; while general hospitals were taken over at the end of the 1930s many of the beds for the sick were still under the jurisdiction of the Poor Law and progress on the implementation of the Local Government Act was slow. Yet there were some municipal general infirmaries quite as well equipped as the voluntary hospitals and a pattern of part-time consultant staffing and of teaching in the hospitals similar to the voluntary hospitals, was under way. Thus the separation of acute and chronic care was maintained and even heightened. Meanwhile, the year 1937 saw a further enquiry by the Hospital Association into the parlous state of the voluntary hospitals; increasingly, the maldistribution and lack of co-ordination between hospitals became clear. The BMA agreed that some scheme of regionalisation was necessary (Abel-Smith 1964).

The 1920s and 1930s therefore saw the emergence of debate about the hospitals and the recognition on the part of many that reorganisation was inevitable. This fact goes a long way towards explaining what was actually to transpire under the 1946 nationalisation act. The hospital sector, including voluntary and local government hospitals, was taken over. Hospitals were nationalised with a clear chain of responsibility from the Ministry through Regional Hospital Boards to Hospital

Management Committees. Early plans for a unified health service however were discarded. The GP service and the Local Authority service with their rivalries and overlaps were left virtually intact. The rueful observation that we got a National Hospital Service not a National Health Service has a great deal of point. The tripartite structure which emerged was a compromise and probably an inevitable one (Stevens 1966; Willcocks 1967; Owen 1968; Eckstein 1958). The matter was reviewed in 1956; the Guillebaud Committee was agreed that the circumstances were not ripe for change (Ministry of Health 1956). In a memorandum of dissent to this Sir John Maude noted two likely consequences of the divided structure as follows:

(a)   the administrative divorce of curative from preventive medicine and of general medical practice from hospital practice and the overlaps, gaps and confusion caused thereby;

(b)   the predominant position of the hospital service and consequent danger of general practice and preventive and social medicine falling into the background . . . (see Owen 1968:6)

Looking back after some twenty years these seem remarkably prescient comments.

The NHS and the Hospitals

It is important to stress that the NHS Act did not in itself emphasise hospital care strongly. In particular it explicitly envisaged, as well as hospital provision, the setting up of health centres. What was planned was that the new national specialist services (i.e. what has become the hospital-based Consultant Service) could be dispensed in such local centres, local authority clinic services could be provided, information and lectures on health could be given and general practitioner and dental services could be available from this site. The health committees of local authorities were empowered to provide such centres as places where, in agreement with executive councils, such services could be dispensed from a single site. What happened was less impressive. In the first ten years of the NHS no further health centres were added to an existing figure of ten (Curwen and Brookes 1969).

The interpretation of pre-NHS history above should render this less than surprising. Health centres were not a new notion, but their exact functions and details of operation remained a fuzzy idea in a context where research and training work had become concentrated in hospitals which themselves were focused on acute care. The arrangements envisaged were ones which required co-operation between GPs and local authorities, two groups which had grown apart after 1911 and, to some extent, become mutually suspicious camps. Furthermore, the new legislation erected additional barriers. Local Authority health committees were left to interpret needs locally; the mechanisms of ministry circular, of building notes as guidelines, of enquiry into particular areas, all mechanisms to effect change in hospitals, were missing in the local authority case. We shall see the results of this below. And finally, no special source of funds was forthcoming for the new enterprise and central government policy turned to other directions. A valuable discussion of these points is available in Etheridge (1976).

The results of creating a clear line of hierarchical control for one sector only, the hospital sector, are clearly revealed in the early 1960s. The year 1962 marked the publication of 'A Hospital Plan for England and Wales' (Ministry of Health 1962). What now emerged was a criticism of separate specialist hospitals and a new policy focused upon the district general hospital (DGH). What is of interest here is not the detail of this plan, but the point that it constituted a full-blown plan for hospital provision. Treatment of other aspects of the health service was significantly different. A document was published on community health services the following year (Ministry of Health 1963). But it comprised a set of targets the Ministry had requested local authorities to provide for their various services and a commentary on the discrepancies between these. The discrepancies were large. No strong initiative was taken giving a lead on the type of non-hospital service which would be preferable. A similar approach was taken to GP services. A report was also made available in 1963 but it was advisory only and concentrated on very broad principles and appeared to be most hesitant about 'interfering' with GPs (see Stevens 1966:249). Interestingly both the Hospital Plan, and what can be seen as an even stronger advocacy of the DGH, the Bonham-Carter Report (Central Health Services Council 1969) are at pains to stress that hospital development was only to be one component of a comprehensive health service for an area. Indeed for some groups the 1962 plan envisaged less hospital provision than had hitherto been available. Separate residential care for many of the subnormal was stressed, and reference made to expansion of community services. The DGH would have an active treatment assessment unit for short-stay geriatric cases and mental illness cases. Again the emphasis was to be on expanding community facilities.

For these reasons, official doctrine, as in 1946, cannot be said to be hospital centred. The tripartite administrative structure with its clearer control of hospitals, however, seems to have generated detailed initiative in that area and rather vaguer exhortations elsewhere. With divisions and overlaps between GPs and LHAs on who was to do what it was not surprising that ideas about primary/community care should stagnate and that patterns of resource allocation already alluded to should take the direction they did.

The last ten years or so, however, have seen much apparent change. First there has been health centre building, taking off from around 1964. Three new centres were opened in that year with a further 26 starting operation between 1964 and 1967. Some 37 were opened in the first nine months of 1969 (Curwen and Brookes 1969). Second, the 1974 Act has brought administrative change and an apparently integrative reorganisation. Third, new statements about priorities for planning are emerging which set lower growth targets for the hospital than for other sectors (see Draper *et al.* 1975). Yet from the point of view of hospital-centred health care the likely extent of these changes can be called into question as the paragraphs below briefly indicate. The case of recent priorities statements will serve to indicate why.

I have selected for examination a document recently emanating from the Department of Health and Social Security on planning priorities (DHSS 1976c). Taken at face value this seems to be so direct an attack on hospital-centredness that the concept in any sense must come under severe challenge. Is this in fact so? A number of recent commentators think not (Klein *et al.* 1974; Klein 1975; Radical Statistics Group 1976; Heller 1978). First there are distinct echoes of an older approach. This is clear in the comment that the primary care sector is 'not susceptible to the same degree of budgetary control as services directly provided by statutory field authorities', and again in reference to 'natural development' in this sector as determined by public demand and professional response. It is also clear in the reference to joint authorities. Local government services in the guise of personal social services are seen as a vital part of provision, yet, given the shape of local government and health administrative reform, joint planning and the older theme of co-ordination survives. Nor does the stress on planning for particular groups, what I shall term 'categorical planning', suggest immediate change — by and large because categorical planning is overlaid with planning of the older type, the very *sectoral planning* which has been shown to be a factor in hospital bias. Can an emphasis on categorical planning effect real change? There are reasons for doubt, for the budgetary reallocations are not as substantial as they may appear. Attention here must be paid to the absolute magnitude of the differences in resource allocation, and to the baseline. Clearly it would take a very long time for these differential growth rates to have a discernible effect on the overall proportions allocated to each sector. Attention should also be paid to the point that much of the expenditure is on manpower and thus difficult to shift without severe disruption for employees. And what when financial crises lessen? We may note a sentence at one point which reads: 'if more resources were available there would be a strong case for increasing the general hospital capital programme . . . '. This is not just sectoral planning co-existing with categorical planning, but the old bias in favour of the hospital sector again. Examples come from those skills, groups and services which are least associated with the hospital, the social workers. Their orientation to care provision is clear in the following passage:

> The philosophy . . . [is] to identify and respond to the differing needs of families and individuals in the community, irrespective of how they arose . . . Families in need of help often present a mixture of problems . . . The personal social services have to decide how to respond to a larger and varied range of problems which are themselves interwoven with forces affecting society more widely. (DHSS 1976c: para. 10.1)

What is important here is the way in which this 'health care' is divorced from the medically oriented programme of the hospital with its focus on the acutely ill, dependent patient. The help needed is not necessarily of any particular sort, it may be preventive or ameliorative, financial, educational and so on. Such a line of thinking, however, emanates from social services departments now firmly outside the health authorities. The client groups identified as in need of special treatment are in part the responsibility of the local authorities. How far hospital-centredness pervades the treatment of client groups may well be a function of the degree to which they come under the control of these two authorities.

This brief example is given to draw attention not only to the very real difficulties at a political and economic level of shifting resources of all kinds when those resources are so massively skewed in a particular direction, but also to problems at the level of conceptualising alternatives. Many things contribute to this. Foremost among them, I suspect, is training. The same processes that concentrated health care practice in the hospital, concentrated training, research and status there too (see Atkinson in this volume). When the first model of disease causation the student meets is the mechanistic one, and when, as in the acute hospital

setting with its selected patients, that model is so self-evidently successful, there is little impetus to talk about alternatives. There is something
else here too. For a long time sociologists have been studying the
training process among doctors and nurses, and arguing that it does
much more than transmit technical knowledge. It inculcates attitudes
and values, and it also reproduces social relations.

The social relations of the hospital include a marked dependency on
the part of the patient, strict and discontinuous hierarchies of hospital
workers, a centrality for the doctor and a control by him over technological resources. (Contrast the position of the patient 'at home' — it is
open to question whether he is clinically ill; he has choices of who to
consult, he has a lay support group in the family. He faces a lower status
doctor (a generalist) and interacts with subordinated health workers
(home nurses, health visitors etc.) on his own ground in perhaps a more
personalised way, without the hierarchical constraints operating on
them in the hospital.) Such relations are not ones in which change is
easily introduced and the studies which clarify these relations have
important lessons for policy makers (Dingwall 1977b; Atkinson 1977;
Bucher and Stelling 1977).

Factors such as these operate in addition to the direct interests some
groups, of course, have in the maintenance of the hospital as a locale
for health delivery. Groups as varied as trade unions and professional
associations may be involved here (see Dingwall in this volume) as well
as the industries which supply the hospital. Direct interests and conceptual blinkers then are factors for investigation in considering
hospital-centred health care, and the parties involved are not
exactly the same as in the past.

Conclusion

The themes of this account are several. We must note that hospitals in
the early nineteenth century existed to serve social control functions
expressed through the charitable impulses of wealthy lay persons, and
through the operation of the Poor Laws. The role of doctors and of
medical knowledge in them was minimal. Later the voluntary institutions were captured by doctors and shaped by the power and interests
of that group to deal with what they defined as interesting cases rather
than to be a resource for the poor. The availability of Poor Law institutions for the rejected helped this process, though later they too via a
rather different dynamic moved in a similar direction. This fed and was
fed by two factors. One was stratification in, and uneven development
of, medical knowledge which legislation of 1911 and 1946 strengthened

more than it challenged. Another was the separation of Local Authority, General Practitioner and hospital services which again found expression in legislation and which the 1946 Act faithfully reproduced. Hospital-centred health care thus came about as a function of development in economic and political structures. Its current persistence however is aided by the accretion of a knowledge base of clinical medicine which arises from and strongly legitimates current arrangements. Hospital-centred health care, in short, has been a policy without a proponent, a bias in the delivery of health care which emerged from and was shaped by the social relations of an earlier era.

It would be idle to deny the benefits of hospital-centred health care and the reality of the advantages which have accrued in the understanding and control of ill health via this particular way of organising resources and of conceptualising disease. But ours is a particularly critical moment for reflection. Back at the setting up of the NHS, we were faced with the growing cost of hospital facilities and the impossibility of meeting that cost in the traditional way. We did not question the need for more hospital facilities then, and now the idea of hospital-centred health care is more firmly embedded. Once again the growing cost of hospitals is its issue. But the context this time is slump not boom, and there is a crisis in state expenditure.

What is the likely result? I would suggest that the following trends are already apparent. The hospital, along with its workers, is being regarded as a more scarce and more central resource such that the only possibility is seen to be to use it highly intensively and selectively. This means waiting lists will lengthen, stays will shorten, costs will be thrown back wherever possible on to the community and the home. Such rationing will produce criticism from many, and the demand for private practice and indeed for private hospitals will increase. Defenders of the NHS will be alarmed at this, but some at least will regard it as acceptable — as a way of protecting the hospital — the inevitably costly *core* of the health service. Health workers, even now convinced of the status and importance of hospital posts, will compete even harder to reach the hospital, the elusive pinnacle of their professions.

We hear a lot about 'community care', 'primary care' and 'treatment' in a 'health service'. These obscure the point that the service is a hospital-centred one. It became hospital centred not via conscious policy decisions but via the interests and activities of the various groups involved. Furthermore, since the hospital is a social institution, it produces and reproduces the skills and social relations necessary for its own survival.

Acknowledgements

This is a revised and shortened version of a paper presented to the European Group on Organisation Studies, Health Organisations Group Conference, Augsburg, 1977. I am grateful to several friends and colleagues for their comments on the original version, namely: David Armstrong, Alan Beattie, Brian Clarke, Michael Carpenter, Arthur Francis, Olgierd Kuty, Tom Manson, Janine Nahapiet, Margaret Stacey and Rex Taylor.

4 THE PRODUCTION OF MEDICAL PRACTITIONERS

Paul Atkinson

Introduction

A consideration of medical education in the context of the National Health Service highlights one recurrent paradox. In Britain the NHS is the major employer of medical manpower — it is virtually a monopolist. The NHS also provides the institutional framework for much medical training at the undergraduate and postgraduate levels. A naïve observer might therefore assume a degree of congruence between the requirements of the National Health Service, and the medical training provided in the United Kingdom. Yet such an assumption would be misleading. There are points at which pains are taken (and inflicted) in the cause of tailoring the production of doctors to the NHS, but there are also numerous points at which discrepancy arises between the two.

Of course, doctors are by no means the only profession who exercise power and influence within the NHS, nor do they enjoy a monopoly of expert knowledge. Nevertheless, the doctors exert a special influence having as they do a dominant position in the provision of health care in general, and the NHS in particular. It is, therefore, of importance to examine how, and in what numbers, doctors are produced. The issue of 'manpower' and the production of medical practitioners may appear to be merely a technical matter. It is all too easy to assume that no more is involved than the accurate production of demographic trends and estimation of future 'needs'. Such calculations are important but they provide only part of the answer. The question of quantity is intimately related to questions of quality: we need to consider not only the number but also the sort of doctors produced. 'Manpower' cannot be divorced from the career structure of the medical profession, nor from the division of labour within it. (For a similar discussion of this issue, at an earlier date, see Stevens 1966.)

The forecasting of the needs for qualified medical practitioners, both in general and in particular specialist fields and across different regions, and the matching of such forecasts with the eventual provision of manpower, exemplify the necessary relation between medical education and the NHS. The intersection of the 'needs' of the NHS and the organisation and structure of medical education has recently shown tensions over such forecasting.

Despite, or perhaps because of, the importance of the forecasting and provision of doctors, the history of such projections has been no happier than that of any other predictions in higher education. The 'inaccuracies' of planning for teacher education have produced bitter controversy in educational and political circles as colleges had to be opened and expanded in the 1960s at great speed, and then equally precipitately cut down and closed in the 1970s. A similarly rancorous argument is building up in medical circles due to equally 'inaccurate' forecasting of the need for medical practitioners in the UK. In its submission to the Royal Commission on the National Health Service, for instance, the British Medical Association 'regards the field of medical manpower as one of the most important topics at which the Royal Commission will be looking'. Manpower has suddenly become a burning issue. As Klein (1977) puts it, 'In one of those sudden mass conversions usually associated with religious revivalism, it has become accepted almost overnight that Britain faces an impending surplus of doctors.'

Like religious revivals, crusades over medical manpower come in fairly regular cycles, and the present panic is one in a series dating back before the inception of the National Health Service. There has been a cycle of reports and policies, based now on fears of a shortage of doctors, now on fears of over-production. The Goodenough Report of 1944, which predated the establishment of the NHS, argued that postwar Britain would need to have a larger output from her medical schools. The average annual output from British medical schools before the Second World War had been about 1,800 doctors entering medicine in the UK. Goodenough concluded that there should be about 2,100 new doctors a year and so the annual intake should rise to 2,500 undergraduates. Eleven years later in 1955, the Willink Report concluded that there was imminent danger of producing a surplus of doctors and argued strongly for a reduction in the intake of the medical schools. By 1964, the output of doctors had fallen below the pre-war levels to 1,500 per annum. However, by 1964 the flow of qualified doctors overseas had become much greater than anyone, including the Willink Committee, had expected. Fears were expressed that Britain was facing an acute shortage of doctors.

With these fears about a shortage of doctors caused by the medical 'brain-drain' at their height, the Labour Government established the Royal Commission on Medical Education under Lord Todd in 1965. Todd reported in 1968 and accepted the fears of a severe shortfall in medical manpower, estimating that in the decade 1966-76, Britain would face a deficit of 10,000 doctors. Their solution was an enlargement of the student body in medical school because a 'substantial increase of output of medical graduates was required without delay' (Royal Commission on Medical Education 1968).

The expansion proposed was from the current 2,600 to 5,000 entrants every year, so that by 1985-89 there would be 4,500 graduates annually entering the medical profession in the UK. Todd argued that this substantial increase should be achieved by expanding the intake of existing medical schools and, more radically, by founding new medical schools. The Labour Government accepted the Todd Report and new medical schools were founded at Southampton, Nottingham and Leicester while intakes at existing schools were increased to levels above those reached before the Willink-inspired reductions.

The Present Debate

Though the predictions about a shortfall of doctors were accepted by the government, the Todd Report has not been fully implemented, due largely to recent cuts in public expenditure. The numbers of students in medical schools, and graduates leaving them, has fallen short of the Todd recommendations. One might expect this failure to implement the recommendations in full to have led to public and professional outcry against the cuts in expenditure. In fact, the reverse has occurred. It has recently been suggested from a variety of sources, within and without the medical profession, that Britain is producing too many doctors. The climate of opinion about medical education seems to be recreating the mood which produced the post-Willink reductions. In particular, fears about a surplus of medical school graduates and the spectre of doctors on the dole have been raised by the Junior Hospital Doctors, by the BMA in general and by some public sector economists.

The possibility of an over-production of medical graduates has been highlighted by the arguments of two health economists that Britain already has a small surplus of doctors, and will shortly have a sizeable excess, which will continue for some time to come. The economists Maynard and Walker (1977) tackle the basis of the Todd Report's predictions and criticise its conclusions. The Todd Report produced both short- and long-term estimates of medical manpower requirements. The short-term estimate covered the period from 1966-1975 — the period of the 10,000 shortfall — while the long-term forecast covered the years from 1976-95. For the 1965-76 estimate, Todd relied on a population growth of 0.8 per cent per annum, and for the long-term on the doctor-patient ratio improving at 1.5 per cent per annum. Both these figures are, Maynard and Walker argue, misleading. The population estimates have already been proved incorrect, due to the falling birth-rate. Todd predicted a UK population of 56.4 million for 1975, but the actual figure was only 54.4 million. Of course, Todd was not alone in producing misleading forecasts; the same figure was used for most government planning in the 1960s. An improvement in the doctor-patient ratio of 1.5 per cent is also questionable.

No such improvement can be guaranteed economically, and so must not be assumed in future calculations. Maynard and Walker are also sternly critical of the expansion in hospital posts since Todd and the failure to rectify regional inequalities, arguing that there are currently 3,500 too many hospital doctors while GP demands have not been met. Over all, they argue that doctor demand and supply were balanced in 1975, and Todd's estimated 10,000 shortfall did not materialise. More seriously still, they argue that based on Todd's own forecasting procedures there will be a surplus of 120 doctors in 1980, while if the 1.5 per cent improvement in the doctor-patient ratio is discounted, the surplus will be the startling figure of 5,520, at a cost of £165 millions.

Rudolf Klein (1977) has recently endorsed the idea of a surplus, although he warns:

> The fact that the balance appears to have changed so dramatically in so short a period should, in itself, act as a warning against over-confident conclusions about what is still very much an uncertain future. There appears to be a very real danger of a manic depressive cycle developing, where medical manpower policy is reversed every ten years or so.

Klein points out that neither the structure of the NHS nor the economic environment are static and fixed for all time – nor indeed are the other factors in the forecasting equations. Klein points out that there are at least five imponderables in any forecast: Britain's economic prospects, the likely career patterns of women doctors, the future intentions of immigrant doctors, the future population of the UK, and, not least, the balance between career and training posts within the NHS.

The medical profession have taken up the apparent threat of a surplus of doctors, and the topic has figured prominently in recent debates, occasioned by the establishment of the Royal Commission. The Commission is being pressed for a review of the manpower requirements and provision. Indeed, the need for such review is seen as so pressing that spokesmen argue that we cannot even wait for the Royal Commission to report before reforms are implemented.

In their draft evidence to the Royal Commission the BMA included a detailed section on medical manpower. They concluded, *inter alia*, that given certain assumptions, there was likely to be a surplus of graduates over required numbers by 1985. 'We are', they continue, 'consequently extremely concerned about the possibility of unemployment in the medical profession. There is no need to emphasize the folly of training doctors at considerable public expense who cannot be employed.'

When the draft evidence was debated, it was argued by spokesmen of the junior hospital doctors that the submission did not 'represent adequately the serious anxieties felt by the representatives of 20,000 junior doctors'. They submitted their own evidence as an appendix to the main BMA document. The junior doctors, on their own calculations, concluded that on current policy, Britain would have 80 per cent more economically active doctors than at present. Since the economic climate would preclude any major increase in expenditure on the Health Service, medical unemployment would be inevitable. The junior doctors therefore recommended that 'the annual output of medical graduates should be reduced to 2,600 by an immediate reduction in medical school intake'. This contrasts with the (known) output of medical graduates of 3,687 in 1981. The junior doctors' document was debated at a special Representative Meeting of the BMA. Some spokesmen wanted the juniors' stronger statement substituted for the original draft evidence: this was defeated, and their paper was accepted as an appendix to the submission.

That the junior doctors were very troubled by the prospects of future manpower was clearly indicated in the report of the debate of their document. One representative was reported as saying that: He was sure there would be a glut of doctors in Britain. It was a deliberate policy of the DHSS to create such a glut, so that they could direct labour; doctors would become members of multidisciplinary teams with no authority but with total responsibility. Too many doctors were being produced. Some of the centres of excellence should be closed down; the intake of medical students in provincial teaching hospitals should be frozen and half the London teaching hospitals closed. Doctors would then be free to do what they were trained to do — treat patients where the patients were.

The junior doctors have drawn an explicit comparison with the colleges of education in painting a picture of future unemployment. Of course, colleges of education are much less powerful institutions than are the medical schools, and the medical profession is in a far stronger position than the teachers. None the less, it is symptomatic of the concern felt by the junior doctors that the parallel should be drawn.

Career Patterns

The junior doctors feel in a particularly vulnerable position in the event of an over-production of medical graduates, and it is not surprising that they are the most vociferous advocates of retrenchment in medical school places. They already feel the pinch by virtue of the present staffing and career structure. The junior hospital doctors experience a 'bottleneck' between the junior, training grades, and posts at consultant level. In their document for the Royal Commission they remark that manpower problems are 'made worse by a chaotic and grossly imbalanced staffing structure so that there are too many doctors in the training grades to allow all who have completed adequate training schedules to get through to established career posts'. Similarly, the BMA submission notes that while the graduates opting for general practice are 'reasonably certain' of becoming principals, without undue delay, those choosing a hospital speciality face a much less certain future.

The problem of the career structure arises in part from a discrepancy between the need for training and the need for patient care. While the junior posts are supposed to be filled for training purposes, the responsibilities for patient care have increasingly fallen on the junior grades. The number of junior posts have grown at a faster rate than have consultant posts. In absolute terms, there are insufficient consultant openings to absorb all the candidates in training. To some extent, the discrepancy between training and career posts has been obscured by the presence of overseas graduates, who were not necessarily committed to a continuing career in Britain at consultant level. But at the present time, the competition is beginning to affect British graduates, who do aim to pursue careers as hospital consultants.

There have been attempts to cope with the problems of staffing structure by the creation of career grades below consultant level. The grade of Medical Assistant was proposed by the Platt Report (1961), although it was greeted with little enthusiasm by the profession. The notion was revived, in a slightly modified manner in the Todd Report (1968), although it was again received with little pleasure. There are, at present, about 1,300 medical assistants, but the profession at large remains hostile to the concept of a sub-consultant career grade. In their submission to the Royal Commission, the BMA state that: 'There must not be a subconsultant grade into which would be forced large numbers of individuals suitable in respect of training and personality for consultant status, but unable to achieve it because of an insufficient establishment of consultant posts relative to those in training grades.'

The offence of the subconsultant grade resides in its anomalous character – in particular the assistant's dependent position. One such assistant has expressed the frustration of medical assistants (Roy-Chowdhury 1977):

> There is discontent not only with emoluments but over the threat to professional dignity. In 1977, it would come as a shock to most fair-minded to know that Medical Assistants have little significant say in the running of their day-to-day professional life . . . They become a hybrid of careerist senior doctor *upstairs* with ill-defined status akin to a junior doctor downstairs.

The subconsultant grade is, therefore, unpopular in so far as it goes against what is seen as the *sine qua non* of full professional status – the right to exercise independent clinical judgement. When the criterion of professional standing and self-esteem is independent of judgement and action, a subconsultant grade is seen as demeaning at a personal level, and its existence as a threat to the collective position of the medical profession.

Given the present career structure in relation to the fear of over-production of doctors it would seem that, in part at least, the problem is not simply one of absolute numbers. It is also a reflection of how medical work, its rewards and its prestige are perceived and evaluated by doctors themselves. We can see this more clearly if we examine the 'shortage' of posts rather more closely.

In some specialties the competition for vacant consultant and senior registrar posts is very strong. In others, the so-called 'shortage special-ties', the ratio of vacancies to applicants is much more favourable to those seeking promotion. At the senior registrar level in particular, the contrast between different specialties is marked (cf. Tables 4.1 and 4.2).

Among the surgical specialties, the pressure for posts is most acute. The DHSS figures show that 'competition is likely to be keenest for posts in plastic surgery, neurosurgery, and cardio-thoracic surgery; and in gynaecology and obstetrics'. Competition is likewise keen for general medicine. In contrast, the pressure for posts in geriatrics is much less and the DHSS estimate that demand will exceed the supply of candi-dates for some years. Likewise, the pressure on posts in anaesthetics is considerably lower than in more popular hospital specialties. It is also

Table 4.1: Recruitment to Consultant Posts, Selected
Specialties (1976)[a]

	Applications[b] per post	Candidates[b] per post	%Overseas graduates	% Women
Anaesthetics	2.2	1.5	21	15
General medicine	6.9	2.2	6	0
General surgery	12.6	3.5	0	0
Geriatrics	4.1	1.8	47	13
Gynaecology and Obstetrics	13.5	3.9	0	6
Mental illness (adult)	7.2	2.4	32	14
Mental illness (child)	1.9	1.6	17	44
Paediatrics	3.8	2.2	14	5
Radiology	2.3	1.2	16	11
Radiotherapy	2.9	1.8	33	33

Notes: [a]Based on sample returns
         [b]Many candidates applied for more than one post
Source: *Health Trends*, 1977, Vol. 9, p. 47.

Table 4.2: Recruitment to Senior Registrar Posts, Selected
Specialties (1976)[a]

	Applications[b] per post	Candidates[b] per post	% Overseas graduates
Anaesthetics	5.2	1.3	17
General medicine	12.5	6.2	0
General surgery	27.4	8.4	27
Geriatrics	4.1	1.5	74
Gynaecology and Obstetrics	18.8	3.4	8
Mental illness (adult)	7.3	3.0	37
Mental illness (child)	3.8	1.5	25
Paediatrics	7.9	3.3	18
Radiology	2.1	1.2	33
Radiotherapy	4.6	1.1	43

Notes: [a]Based on sample returns
         [b]Many applicants applied for more than one post
Source: *Health Trends*, 1977, Vol. 9, p. 47.

notable that in the specialties enjoying little popularity, the proportion of overseas-trained doctors recruited tends to be highest. This pattern is repeated for women at consultant level: the proportion of women tends to be highest in the specialties enjoying least popularity.

To some extent the shortages may be artefacts of different rates of expansion in the different specialties; those which have expanded most rapidly in recent years having the apparent shortages, as demand outstrips available numbers of suitably qualified candidates. This may be a contributory factor, yet it is clear that they also reflect the general patterns of popularity and prestige within the medical profession.

It has been repeatedly demonstrated, for instance, that there are very clear differences in popularity between specialties among medical students. Specialties such as medicine (including cardiology and neurology), surgery, obstetrics and gynaecology and paediatrics are marked high in students' career preferences, while other, apparently less glamorous, specialist fields, attract few students. The pattern of students' career ambitions has remained fairly stable over past years, and there is no evidence of any major shifts in medical students' attitudes. Among the hospital specialties the 'shortage' areas are those 'Cinderella' fields which attract few students as the career of their choice.

It is clear that our present system of medical education produces graduates who are typically unwilling to work in many specialist fields. The emphasis of medical education leads them inexorably towards the high-technology hospital specialties in surgery and medicine (such as cardiology), and away from the 'shortage specialties' in the hospital service, or community and occupational medicine (see Gregory in this volume). For many of them even general practice is seen as a poor substitute for the highly regarded hospital specialties. This is hardly surprising. In the great majority of our medical schools the emphasis of clinical teaching is placed overwhelmingly on the diagnosis and treatment of acute illness in the teaching hospital (see Davies in this volume). Although the medical curriculum has undergone considerable change in recent years, its overall impact on the medical undergraduate has remained much the same. The novice learns first and foremost to think in terms of well-defined 'diseases' and their treatment – either by chemotherapy or surgery. The relatively 'messy', inconclusive picture of health and illness in the community is not comprehended within this conceptual framework. Similarly, such fields as mental illness and geriatric medicine conform poorly to the models of acute disease, treatment and cure which are dominant in medical schools and their curricula. Recent changes in the curriculum of British medical schools have included shifts towards greater emphasis on the less favoured specialties, 'community medicine', and general practice. The introduction of the 'behavioural sciences' (sociology and psychology) can be seen as potentially subversive to the prevailing medical model. To some extent they are. Yet the impact of these innovations is minimal in comparison with the still overwhelming effects of entrenched medical paradigms (see Murcott in this volume). In many ways, however, the 'behavioural sciences' are treated as a further adjunct to medical technology, reinforcing rather than undermining the status quo.

It would be rash to fall in too readily with the view of the profession that we are in danger of over-producing doctors, and simply reduce the number of students admitted to British medical schools, and hence the number of qualified graduates produced. The problem is not simply a matter of absolute numbers. As we have seen, the career structure, and doctors' attitudes towards professional practice and status, are implicated. The BMA clearly want every doctor to become a consultant (or a principal GP), and advocate an expansion in the number of posts at that level, as well as a restriction in output. Such an aspiration is implied by doctors' views as to the necessity of 'independent clinical judgement'. But there is no inherent necessity for all doctors to practise medicine in this way.

Admittedly, the attempts to introduce a subconsultant career grade have not met with great success. This is understandable: the very designation 'subconsultant', is unfortunate, as is the title 'medical assistant'. But the problem arises by virtue of the sharp contrast between consultants and non-consultants – between career specialists and trainees – between independent practice and supervised experience. What is needed in the long run is the radical reconstruction of career posts in general. We need a medical profession in which full independence is not the *sine qua non* of status and self esteem (any more than all university academics can demand to become professor as of right). In a sense, it is not the existence of a National Health Service nor the activities of the DHSS which are odd in Britain; nor is the medical assistant the real anomaly. It is the consultant who is the anomaly, in terms both of the existence of a National Health Service, and of the nature of modern health care in general. One of the doctors quoted above complained that the DHSS was bent on making doctors 'members of multidisciplinary teams with no authority but with total responsibility'. This may or may not be deliberate policy, but it would not be the disaster that doctor implied – provided, perhaps, that the medical profession would give up some of the burden of total responsibility.

In fact, a reorganisation of medical care will be implied even by a restriction of student members. If we do remove the present confusion between 'training' and medical care, then the position of specialists themselves will be changed. At present, the consultants can rely on a 'reserve army' to act as junior members of their teams, who take a major responsibility for day-to-day care. If this 'cushion' is to be removed in the future then the consultants (or their equivalents) will have to undertake much more of this routine work – a development of considerable consequence for the future image of the hospital specialist. Alternatively, it may prove necessary for this day-to-day medical work to be delegated to paramedical workers of various sorts. If this second course were to be pursued, then such workers would be unlikely to accept present conceptions of the medical division of labour; they would (reasonably) demand less clear-cut demarcations between doctors and other health workers. The present state of medical dominance would be under assault. In any event, the question of numbers must lead directly towards the redefinition of medical practice and authority. At present, the medical profession's call for a restriction in numbers is unrelated to such a reconceptualisation. Rather, they seem to be arguing in favour of the continuation of an exclusive and dominant position within the hospital sector of health care. The medical spokesmen are haunted by the fear that a surplus of doctors will allow the DHSS to direct medical labour into the less popular specialties and regions. This they regard as an indefensible interference with their professional freedom. Yet they invite state intervention on a massive scale to ensure the preservation of their current position.

Manpower and Womanpower

The expansion of numbers among the medical profession has been accompanied by an increase in the proportion of women recruited. At present the proportion of students entering medical schools is about 40 per cent; in 1968 the Royal Commission reported the proportion as 25 per cent. On the basis of the trend of recent years, women will comprise an increasingly large proportion of the medical profession. The growing representation of women in the profession has become a major factor in the current debate on 'manpower' (and the sexism of the terminology is not insignificant!) and the career structure.

The critical thing which is normally taken as a factor in forecasting staffing needs is the degree of 'wastage' implied by a given proportion of women graduates. Essentially there are two types of 'wastage'. First, there is 'complete wastage' – which accounts for those who emigrate, work in another profession or cease to work altogether. Secondly, there is wastage which stems from long-term but no permanent withdrawal from medical work. The 'wastage' of women tends to be of the second type. Most surveys of the employment patterns of women doctors have shown that, at any given time, about 30 to 45 per cent are working full-time, and another 35 to 40 per cent working part-time. (The problem of 'wastage' among male doctors has received much less attention, though they are more likely than women to be lost to overseas countries or other occupations.)

Women are concentrated in particular specialties within the medical profession as a whole. They are over-represented in the so-called 'shortage specialties', and under-represented in the fields where pressure for jobs is greatest — especially among the surgical specialties. Women also tend to be over-represented in subconsultant career posts, and correspondingly under-represented at consultant level. In many ways, women and overseas doctors are in similar positions — both categories being over-represented among the least popular areas of medicine and in 'second-best' career posts.

Women doctors face difficulties in establishing satisfactory career patterns — married women with children particularly. Their domestic and professional commitments are conventionally seen as conflicting, and their difficulties reflect the sexual division of labour in society in general. Two patterns have been proposed for women's careers in medicine: the development of part-time training and employment, and a discontinuous career, with a break for those bringing up small children. The latter course is highly unsatisfactory, as it is very hard to build and maintain a career with a period of 'time out' — especially in a field which is changing and developing rapidly. The development of part-time employment has, to some extent, helped to further women's careers in medicine. But it has also served to confirm their subordinate status. The expansion of part-time employment has taken place in the 'women's', shortage specialties — again reflecting and reinforcing the sexual stratification of medical specialties. As Elston (1977) has pointed out:

> The attitude to 'part-time' work in medicine is ambiguous. When done by women it is often seen as failure to utilise fully their state-provided training. For the consultant, on the other hand, it may be the hallmark of success enabling him (or occasionally her) partially to opt out of the state-funded service.

While the former is seen as 'wastage' the latter is not. But it is arguable that the availability of women to work part-time generates a supply of labour for the less popular specialties, for under-financed areas. As Elston remarks, 'analysis of the horizontal distribution of women doctors suggests that several branches of medicine are dependent on this under-utilisation (in terms of both the nature of the work and hours)'.

In the context of a 'surplus' of doctors the position of women is
vulnerable. The BMA and their spokesmen believe that every hospital
doctor should have the opportunity to become a fully independent
specialist (i.e. a consultant). Yet it is clear that this is not so even at the
present. As Elston points out the NHS resembles a dual labour market
– that is a market within which:

1. There is a more or less pronounced division into higher paying
   and lower paying sectors.
2. Mobility across the boundary of those sectors is restricted.
3. Higher paying jobs are linked into promotional or career ladders,
   while lower paid jobs offer few opportunities for vertical movement.
4. Higher paying jobs are relatively stable, while lower paid jobs are
   unstable.

In the context of a professional group such as medicine, while pay is
important, distinctions of status and independence may be of equal
importance. At present, women and overseas graduates find themselves
disproportionately in the relatively lowly 'secondary' sector of the
health service market. To that extent they provide a mechanism whereby the number of jobs and the number of available personnel can be
matched, existing as they do as a 'reserve army' of the underemployed
or unpromoted.

The junior doctors are pressing for a reduction in numbers to ensure
satisfactory career prospects. While they note the special position of
women, they do so only in order to calculate the appropriate level of
'wastage'; they do not appear to have come to terms with the nature of
the dual labour market. The aspirations of (male) junior doctors should
not be realised only at the expense of their female counterparts,
through a rigidly divided profession of first- and second-class doctors.

While a reduction in the number of medical graduates could in
theory improve the career prospects of women doctors, there is little
prospect of that in practice. A reduction in numbers alone will not of
itself ensure a more equitable division of labour and enhanced career
prospects for women. Estimates of future staffing needs from all
quarters continue to assume high levels of 'wastage', and so in turn
assume that women will continue to occupy part-time positions.
Women are poorly represented, numerically speaking, among the
spokesmen and politicians of the profession: their interests continue to
be poorly served. Recognition of their potential contribution, and the

efficient use of their labour, coupled with the satisfaction of their career aspirations, will not follow simply from 'manpower' planning; it will require a thorough reappraisal of the career structure.

Conclusion

The parallel between the teachers and the doctors is an obvious one, but it must be used with caution. The recent closure of teacher-training colleges and severe cutbacks in student-teacher numbers cannot be treated as self-evident support for restricting medical school places. While demographic changes affect both, the fall in birth-rate does not have the same immediate consequences for the two professions. Whereas the education system is related directly to changes in the age-structure, medicine is not affected so directly. Indeed, the implications of an ageing population are not such as to reduce the need for health care: if anything the reverse is true.

In any case it is apparent that medicine has not necessarily responded to changes in the birth-rate. One might reasonably expect, for instance, that a falling birth-rate since 1964 would be reflected in the staffing levels and costs of paediatric services. But between 1963 and 1976 — precisely the period when the numbers of children born and growing up were falling — the number of whole-time equivalent staff in paediatrics in England rose from 450 to 1,313. In itself, of course, this is not a bad thing, although it does reflect how contemporary medicine has a momentum of its own, that 'nice inflation' which Cochrane refers to. Falling numbers of children, and a steady growth in the numbers of specialists, could be the opportunity for a major improvement in health care, and the recent Court Report on child health has argued precisely that. Whether or not the continued growth of paediatrics will result in commensurate improvements in health and medical care, the example highlights the fact that medicine is not dependent on the birth-rate or the overall size of the population. In the last analysis, the determination of doctor-patient ratios and the relative priority given to different specialties are political issues; and while demographic trends must be taken into account, they are not the only consideration. To return to the case of the teaching profession, the reduction in training and employment of teachers has not rested solely on the numbers of children of school age. The apparent 'surplus' of teachers has not, for instance, resulted in the reduction of class sizes. The decisions have been economic and political, and not determined by blind demographic trends alone.

If the output of doctors is to be restricted, then we must recognise that this too will be a political and economic decision. Klein (1977) suggests that if Britain 'has become a static, non-growth society' then we must have 'a policy of medical manpower contraception'; if economic growth returns, he argues, this will not necessarily be the case. Klein makes the further point that an increase in the total number of doctors does not necessarily imply an equivalent rise in the cost of health care: it is not the actual number of doctors and their salaries, but also the costs of the treatments and tests prescribed. Klein suggests that if GP lists were reduced, and if GPs had longer to spend with their patients, they might prescribe fewer drugs, make fewer hospital referrals and order fewer tests. In the long run, an increase in the number of GPs could result in a decrease in the overall health bill. That this argument would not apply to hospital doctors, further emphasises the fact that we cannot conduct the argument only about *numbers*: what is important is the number of doctors of different sorts.

It is not possible to conclude this chapter with any single prescription for the future planning of medical manpower. There is no simple conclusion, because the problem is not of that sort. I have tried to indicate that while a 'crisis' in the medical profession is being presented in terms of a problem of 'manpower', the answers (if there are any) are not to be found simply in terms of the absolute numbers of medical graduates produced each year. In the first place, there is no necessary reason why a falling birth-rate and a declining population should result in a reduction in medical personnel — if we were able and willing to pay for the training and employment of such 'extra' doctors, to shorten the waiting lists and reduce GPs' lists. (We could have gone on employing more teachers and finally made a significant reduction in the average size of classes.) On the other hand, there is no guarantee that the doctors produced would be deployed to the best effect — either in terms of their regional distribution, the specialties they pursue or the treatments they prescribe. The national health could be better served by a smaller number of doctors working more efficiently, and with a much greater emphasis on the promotion of health.

We have seen that present concern over manpower has been precipitated by problems of the career structure and promotion prospects for junior hospital doctors. Obviously this is a real and pressing problem for the staff concerned. But the solution does not lie simply in tailoring future numbers to the present structure. In the long term, the development of health care is not facilitated by preserving the out-moded distinction between the independent consultant and his own firm of subordinates. We should move towards the abolition of this bipartite division of the hospital service. More suited to the needs of the hospitals and the nature of modern health care would be the creation of a general, 'specialist' career, with the abolition of the present rigid division, and a series of subgrades. There would be no necessary assumption of full independent practice, nor the corresponding stigma of the sub-consultant grade.

A reduction in the number of doctors will be welcome if it results in a radical reappraisal of priorities for medical employment. A retrenchment is to be resisted if it serves only the restrictionist interests of a profession committed to the present state of affairs, with its maldistribution of doctors, and the existing career patterns. By the same token, we must ask whether, in advocating a reduction, the medical profession will accept changes in the division of labour. That is, whether the demand for doctors is to be reduced by allocating more work to other, 'paramedical' professions (nurses, pharmacists etc.) (see Austin, Eaton and Webb in this volume), or whether they seek to preserve their position as a small elite group within the health field.

The medical profession, in their submission to the Royal Commission, have called for a new approach to manpower planning. Rather than the past pattern — a review every ten years or so — they demand the establishment of an 'independent review body', routinely to monitor the production of medical personnel. Certainly the pattern of recent decades has proved unsatisfactory on many counts, and the manic swings of over- and under-estimating should not be repeated. But as I have tried to indicate, the issues involved go far beyond numbers alone. The attempt to hive off medical manpower from the political arena, and to portray the issues simply as technical problems of accurate forecasting, should be resisted. We are dealing with crucial questions of the economics and politics of health care, and the debate must be joined in that light.

Acknowledgements

I should like to thank my fellow editors for their helpful comments, and Sara Delamont for her help and encouragement in the preparation of this essay.

5 THE FAILURES OF HEALTH EDUCATION

Muir Gray and Max Blythe

Introduction

Health education is one of the major arms of preventive medicine. It has gained favour as investment in curative medicine has yielded diminishing returns and caused an increasing amount of side-effects and iatrogenic disease. The last decade has seen a considerable development of health education in the National Health Service and in the education system.

Despite its increasing popularity the whole conception of health education remains confused. In the first place there is confusion over the nature of 'health'. Asked to define health in a single sentence most people would probably offer something like the World Health Organisation's definition: 'complete physical, social and mental wellbeing . . . '. Few realise that the definition continues:' . . . not merely the absence of disease or infirmity'. The failure to recognise this is the cause of many of the problems of health education. In fact it has been, and remains in many quarters, almost exclusively *illness* education.

There is, too, confusion over the place of health education in the school curriculum. Where it does feature it appears as a specialist, separate subject, whereas, we believe, it should be a theme running through the whole curriculum. Given the current demand for examinable school subjects, the place of health education remains unsure.

Health Education and Health Professions

Many health professionals still see treatment as a process separate from education. Yet education and treatment are, inevitably, closely related. If communication is ineffective, then so is treatment. It has, for instance, been shown that non-compliance with medication is very frequent, and that compliant behaviour can only occur as a result of appropriate communication (e.g. Hulka *et al.* 1976). Many doctors now accept that Aesculapean authority is not enough to ensure effective communication, though there is still a strong belief that doctors can teach by virtue of the fact that they are doctors. It is mostly in the newer medical schools that time is found in the curriculum for ideas which might make students better communicators and educators. The only branches of medicine in which health education plays an integral

89

part are rehabilitation, health visiting, midwifery, some branches of psychiatry and the new style of general practice.

Very little is known about professionals' attitudes towards health education. However, a recent paper on 'Smoking and Professional People' (DHSS 1977a) reveals that the majority of professionals feel they ought to discourage people from smoking: from 70 per cent of pharmacists up to 86 per cent of hospital doctors. Interestingly, the report mentions that there was a 'strong tendency' for professionals to 'see their role in anti-smoking education as one of encouraging smokers, particularly patients with smoking-related diseases, to stop smoking. There was less frequent mention of encouraging people not to start smoking.' (Midwives and health visitors were exceptions, seeing both aspects as their responsibility.) Many professionals, then, appear to hold rather limited conceptions of health education, while it remains marginal to much medical work. There are signs that attitudes are changing: a number of doctors and primary care teams are taking a more educative approach. But skills are often lacking, and we are still some way off the development of *health* professions.

Health Education in Schools

Health education in schools is experiencing change, reappraisal and reformation. This development is by no means premature. For too long the subject's image has been one of narrowly based health warnings, concerned with the facts about germs, sex, drugs and smoking. Its scope rarely extended so far as to allow pupils the opportunity to discuss personal and social perspectives, or the experience of decision making. Although there have been changes, there are still important barriers to progress: entrenched attitudes within the teaching profession, confusion over the nature of health education, disagreement over the status of a subject too wide and diffuse to fit neatly into a subject-based curriculum.

Today's changes have their origins in the 1960s and early 1970s. In 1964 the Cohen Committee on Health Education provided some major recommendations. The report made clear the need for a broadly based health education syllabus in schools, aimed at 'giving the child such knowledge as will equip him to face the social and health problems he will meet in later years'. Influential though this report was, nevertheless it still retained something of an illness orientation.

Perhaps the major stimulus towards education for health has come from the curriculum developments sponsored by the Schools Council, the Health Education Council, and the Nuffield Science Project Team.

One of the most significant developments likely to influence attitudes to the subject has been the establishment of the project 'Health Education 5-13' by the Schools Council. This has emphasised the view that health education should lay essential foundations in the earliest years of a child's school career. The development of this project has involved a substantial cross-section of interests in health education and the links established may well prove to be the most influential aspect of the whole enterprise. A further, complementary project, 'Health Education 13-18' is under way, in search of 'ways in which health education can be organized within a secondary school curriculum' and the development of support materials.

In 1976 the Schools Council Working Party, in 'Working Paper 57' expressed its views on health education in secondary schools. It sought to help heads and assistant teachers organise health education in ways appropriate to the special requirements of their schools, stressing that each school must research and plan its own approach.

Working in tandem with the Schools Council has been the Health Education Council, which serves as a watchdog over the many interests in health education in England, Wales and Northern Ireland. (Scotland has its own excellent Health Education Unit.) The Council's responsibilities are outlined in its annual report. They are: to advise on priorities for health education; to advise and carry out national, and occasionally local, campaigns; to produce information and publicity material in support of campaign interests; to undertake and sponsor research; to seek advice and review relevant literature; to act as a national centre of expertise; to encourage and promote training in health education work. The Council's responsibility, then, is to set the climate in which health education can evolve.

In the last two years have come other important contributions to the published debate. The Department of Health and Social Security raised its voice in 'Prevention and Health: Everybody's Business' (DHSS 1976a). That paper outlines 'how much depends upon the attitudes and actions of the individual about his health'.

In principle there is impressive and widespread support for the current developments. But real progress awaits the translation of good-will into effective practice in the schools. Admittedly these are early days in which to assess the response of the schools, but there are several significant questions that can be raised: What has happened in teacher-training establishments? What status does the subject enjoy? Has there been a significant change in the allocation of special responsibility payments to specialist teachers? How far have schools and colleges pro-

gressed towards the introduction of a broadly based curriculum for all
age groups and ability ranges?

The answers to these questions are disappointing. Given the current
response in teacher-training colleges, the provision of posts and responsibility allowances, and limited curriculum developments, health education in schools is unlikely to experience even reasonable rates of expansion. There is enthusiasm and support for health education in schools
and colleges, but there are considerable barriers to actual achievement.

Health Education – Why Is It Failing?

Before evaluating health education one point must be made in its
defence. The time-scale over which it might be effective is great –
decades rather than years, generations rather than cohorts – and any
effects are hard to measure. Even when change can be detected, health
education is only one of many possible factors. In some senses, then,
health education is in a 'no-win' position. If no effect can be measured
it is said to have failed; if change is demonstrated the critics of health
education can attribute it to other influences. We must keep this in
mind in our appraisal of health education.

Confusion is inherent in the evolution of educational method; it is
a stimulus to thought. But where confusion is unresolved it can become
a major barrier to reform, and this is the case in health education. The
trend away from the traditional approach – hygiene, diet and sex – has
robbed teachers of a clear-cut method. Health education is no longer
seen as a one-way flow of accepted facts from the teachers to the pupils.
The trend is towards a spirit of social inquiry.

Modern health education seeks to examine behavioural patterns and
processes of decision making which determine the health and survival of
individuals and societies. It is about personal and social perspectives,
and its approach is based on a wide range of interests rather than fear of
disease. That being 'healthy' is less about a few facts and figures on
disease than about a much broader preparation for life is the core of
current attitudes. Health education is no longer a subject or a branch of
any other discipline. It has to be incorporated in many different parts
of the curriculum, which creates difficulties and slows progress. However, it is not enough to consider health education solely in the context
of the curriculum. Bernstein (1975) has distinguished between the
'instrumental order' of the school – where health education is normally
found at present – and the 'expressive order', which is concerned with
conduct, character and manner. We believe that the present confusion
can be resolved only when health education is firmly rooted in the ex-

pressive order, the ethos of the whole school.

Resistance in Education

In the context of the so-called Great Debate, education is being judged by its ability to inculcate examinable skills. In such a climate health education is unlikely to compete successfully for curriculum opportunities against subjects offering more *kudos* in public examinations. Even where a headteacher is willing to contemplate such a change there may be resistance from parents, governors and public. Parents anxious about their children's career prospects may find it hard to support an increased commitment to health education if it is at the expense of formal qualifications, for University, College, or apprenticeships. In our experience, a significant proportion of parents consider health education an unnecessary aspect of school life, believing that the home is the right and proper place for it.

Opposition is also encountered from teachers who believe that the best health education is an unseen and non-quantifiable element in the day-to-day partnership between teachers and pupils; that at its best it is a natural rapport that no amount of planning can engineer. There are also some teachers who resist any innovation which might erode the numbers of pupils taking their own subject, and hence threaten their professional status. Even where health education finds support in a school, often there is no consensus over who should teach what, when, and to which pupils. In many schools, however, the main barriers remain those of inertia and indifference.

The Cultural Barrier

The health education movement is drawn largely from Social Classes I and II. Those who are most often ill, and who have shown least response to health education, are mainly in the lower social classes. This is illustrated dramatically in the prevalence of smoking. In 1974 only 27 per cent of men and 21 per cent of women in Social Class I smoked; among unskilled manual workers the figures were 65 per cent and 47 per cent respectively. This is a gap which has recently widened. It has been suggested that the professional advice is often rejected solely because it comes from higher social classes. But in our opinion this is not the reason. We believe that much of the failure can be accounted for by cultural — particularly linguistic — differences.

The vocabulary of health education is now carefully chosen and many semantic misunderstandings have been ironed out. But the linguistic system, the grammar, in which the messages are set is too often incomprehensible. Those health educators who have translated their messages for immigrant groups are to be congratulated, but those who use English should also think of translating their messages into the vernacular. They are written in Standard English, which is but one of many varieties of spoken English (Strange 1962). Health education uses language in which the future and conditional tenses are prominent, because it stems from professionals who live in a culture in which a long-term future is real. Professionals have postponed the end of their education and the onset of earnings in the interests of their future. They live in homes mortgaged for twenty years. They have jobs which are secure, pensioned and superannuated. They have usually been brought up in homes where the same perceptions of future time were present and could be learned. Those in the lower social classes more often live in accommodation rented by the week and work in jobs which could end at short notice. They have usually been brought up in the same culture, marked by what Hoggart (1958) has described as the 'immediacy' of working-class life.

Health education offers a possible gain for the future, twenty or thirty years hence, if present gratification is postponed. Those in the health education movement must realise that the apparent illogicality of wanting to be free of pain and disability, while continuing to behave in a way which predisposes to them, is rational given the linguistic and cultural context in which such decisions are made. If the future is inconceivable beyond next Friday, the present gratification will be preferred (see also Miers in this volume).

Health education has failed whenever it has assumed that there is only one culture in Britain. Even when its message can be understood, however, it is often ignored for reasons it is unable to take into account. It is often assumed that people welcome the opportunity to take over responsibility for their health from the medical profession. But this assumption is unwarranted. Since the birth of scientific medicine doctors have steadily assumed all knowledge and responsibility for the management of illness. In the last few years this has been running into the sand, as the limits of medicine have been more widely recognised. To the great discomfort of many patients, doctors have started to explain that they cannot always diagnose what is wrong. Conditioned to a diagnosis and a bottle, the patients feel very unprotected. The medical profession now tells the public that its fate lies very much in its own control. Faced with this awesome responsibility many prefer to believe in chance — that 'there is a bullet with my number on it', or 'my grandfather lived till eighty, smoking forty a day'.

Health and freedom from illness are high priorities, but fear of illness and recognition of one's frailty are low. Better to allow fantasy freedom, and to trust in fate, rather than listen to the advice of health educators. While it persuades some to act, the worry and anxiety created by health education is too much for many people.

There are further barriers to health education. A person may imagine the future, comprehend the message of health education, and accept that his behaviour increases the risk of illness. But he may continue with his risk behaviour becuase its social significance is of higher priority than its medical significance. Action which appears irrational to the health educator may be rational when viewed from a different social perspective.

This is particularly relevant to health education in adolescence. As Miers (in this volume) discusses at length, adolescence is a period of transition during which rules are broken in the search for a separate identity. Forbidding a certain type of risky behaviour presents an opportunity for the adolescent to become deviant. Risk plays an important role in the *rite de passage* of adolescence.

What opportunities have young people for danger in our society other than crime, action on the terraces, or behaviour which health educators might identify as dangerous? Longevity has little appeal for young people. Death does not provide much fear, provided it is quick; not only because the young people cannot conceive of the future, but because death is seen as an alternative to old age. The future is shrinking for young people as unemployment looms increasingly on the school-leaving horizon. How much attention can health education expect, discussing preparation for the future when the rest of education offers no more than weekly signing-on as a reward for successful completion? The answer is very little, even if health educators have the courage to discuss this paradox with young people, and none if they do not, which is the common approach at present. Illness is not only a physical but a social condition and health education must consider the culture in which people live and become ill. Health education is mono-cultural in its approach, dominated by a limited set of values.

The Ethical Barrier

There was ethical opposition to preventive medicine in the nineteenth century based on a number of principles, prominent among which was J.S. Mill's classic statement in 'On Liberty' – 'The only purpose for which power can rightfully be excused over any member of a civilised society is to prevent harm to others.' Opposition to preventive medicine is still prevalent, the resistance to fluoridation and seat belt legislation being among the most publicised examples. It is probable that this resistance will grow, as a protest not only against the infringement of freedom but against the increasing amount of legislation and consequent centralisation. There is also growing opposition to health education on ethical grounds which not all health educators appear to have realised.

Government and health educators have moved away from attempts to educate by the creation of fear, motivated, perhaps, less by ethical reasons than by a growing awareness that such an approach was of limited effectiveness. There has also been a welcome appreciation of the ethical implications of education which creates guilt, for example, the possibility of creating guilt in pregnant women who smoke by publicising the association between cigarette smoking and low birth weight. However, little consideration has been given to the ethical issues raised by health education as a whole.

As health education has shifted from an approach intended to be informative to one designed to be influential, it has turned its attention to changing attitudes and values directly, by means other than by the presentation of facts. Government agencies and agents which attempt this are engaged in an activity which is more akin to propaganda than to education. A propagandist approach may be justifiable when industry is using the same methods to a much greater extent, but this is an issue which requires much more public discussion if suspicion and resistance are not to flourish.

Ways, Means and Ends

When reviewing prescriptions for health education, it is tempting to concentrate on ways and means to the exclusion of debate about the ends in view. Ways and means are of course important and there are certain structural and organisational changes in professional training or public services concerned with health education which we consider necessary. Here, by way of example, we deal with six such proposals.

First, we recommend the nomination of a Parliamentary Under Secretary in the Department of Health and Social Security as Minister with special responsibility for preventive medicine. We think that there should be a Junior Ministers' Preventive Medicine Committee drawing together the interests of the Departments of Education, Environment, Employment, Sport, and the Treasury, in an integrated approach to preventive medicine which also includes health education.

Second, the Social Science Research Council (SSRC) should be asked to take over responsibility for research conducted by academic departments and special research teams. The SSRC has already considered further commitments in the health field, for example in research on cigarette smoking. We believe that the institution of an SSRC health education research unit would provide a much needed boost. The brief to the SSRC should be to concentrate in particular on attitudes to risk, professional attitudes and behaviour and communication issues in preventive medicine. Opportunities for research should be extended beyond the more usual academic boundaries to encourage contributions from field workers. A small school-based research project should qualify for support just as much as the work of a highly specialised team, in that results from both are significant contributions to the same spectrum of knowledge. A great deal of research is already being conducted in Britain, for example in Leeds, Manchester and Nottingham, but the overall research effort must be more rigorously stimulated and controlled if effectiveness and efficiency is to be improved. The Scottish Health Education Unit has shown the kind of approach which should be taken (Tones 1977) in order to provide the much needed strengthening of the empirical foundations of health education.

Third, we think it is essential that steps be taken to guarantee adequate resources for health education at local level. It is useless for the Department of Health to express the hope that health authorities will develop health education unless it ensures that they receive sufficient resources to do so. This could be done using the Health Education Council as 'banker'. Indeed, the Council has already pioneered a step in this direction. Some of the extra money allocated to the Council is being used to train Health Education Officers whose employing authorities could not find the money for it. This is one way in which central intentions can be implemented in the periphery. Another is for Health Authorities to develop contingency funds to meet the cost of new ideas in preventive medicine. Even such well-proven measures as screening to detect spina bifida (alpha-fetoprotein screening is known to be effective) find the competition for resources difficult when the demands of the acute services, themselves in straitened circumstances, are set against them. Long-term savings with a wide range of benefits and economies in the provision of services have little appeal. The health education pay-off is not only in the distant future, it is also hard to prove. Health education can only hope for resources if Health Authorities save a small amount, perhaps of the order of one quarter of one per cent from every budget, for a pump-priming fund both for health education and for those clinical services which can prevent disability and pain.

Fourth, it is important to clarify and make adequate provision for supporting the work of the country's Health Education Officers. Although there are now several hundred of them, their influence is limited by various factors: the lack of a coherent identity, variable levels of staffing and support finance and the need to work in education although located outside the education system itself. Within the present national provision we continue to find examples of Area Health Authorities which have been dilatory in appointing Health Education Officers, and others which have made appointments, but to posts with inadequate budgets. This will not get us very far. Each Area Health Authority must accept its share of the national responsibility, making clear its aims and the resources essential to the agreed strategy. Representatives of the Health Education Council could play a major part in helping to co-ordinate the overall national approach. Theirs could be the task of linking related interests and developing a pool of experience. To date, whether by accident or by design the approach of Health Education Officers has tended to be separatist. Health Education practice is a research frontier and progress demands more effective liaison between the various teams of officers working at field level. Health Education Officers themselves perhaps hold the major key to the success of their interest. Much depends upon the skill with which they handle 'middle man' status and/or the strength of their original contributions to research and education. A distinct identity for the new occupation of Health Education Officer is not likely to develop from a 'middle man' role of conveying information from texts they did not write to a public they have not researched.

Fifth, Local Education Authorities (LEAs) must also accept a greater share of responsibility. If the current health education input of the Schools Council and Health Education Council's curriculum projects is to flourish, there must be good local preparation for schools. In the spirit of recent initiatives, the former Chief Education Officer for Oxfordshire has said 'Each school needs its own health education programme, and every teacher must know about the school's scheme of work and his own involvement in it' (DHSS 1977b). Such a goal is only realistic if LEAs are prepared to sponsor substantial advisory contributions and provision of support materials. Many teachers are frightened by aspects of health education which they know are controversial and most of them lack the 'enlightened' background we believe ought to stem from teacher-training courses. LEAs must clarify their priorities and then fund advisory and resource services accordingly. Many of them might consider closer liaison with their Area Health Authorities and

local health education services. One way could be to follow the
example of East Sussex and Oxfordshire where Health Education Co-
ordinators have been jointly appointed by the AHA and the LEA, with
the aim of encouraging close collaboration of educationalists and AHA
personnel.

Sixth, a national review of the role, distribution, staffing and
training needs of health visiting is long overdue (Dingwall 1977).
Health visiting is pulled in different directions by conflicting interests;
towards children, towards old people, towards preventive medicine and
towards social casework. The problem of what health visiting itself
should be, urgently requires resolution. The Council for the Education
and Training of Health Visitors has produced a useful booklet raising
fundamental questions about the nature of health visiting (Council for
the Education and Training of Health Visitors 1977). The Department
of Health should use this as a basis for a complete review of the profession's future.

A new subject or theme can never grow and flourish in education
while the whole field is felt to be contracting and morale is low. In
those parts of the country where education and other public services
have been hard hit by the loss of rate support grants and schools have
had to lose staff, headteachers have had a difficult enough task maintaining those school departments already established. In those areas
which are said to have benefited from this shift in resources, the
schools have had other problems to face in supporting and containing a
juvenile population disillusioned by the prospect of impending unemployment. Any beneficial effects of the transfer of rate support grant
have been neutralised by the social problems faced by the city schools.
Health education can itself only flourish in a healthy environment.
Until the government realises that education for less-talented young
people between the ages of 12 and 25 requires a massive injection of
funds, even, if necessary at the expense of higher education, health
education will fail to prosper.

We believe, however, that too much faith is placed in reorganisation
and structural change, which risks losing sight of the ends to be
achieved. The debate should be about the objectives of health education. Rather than the broad approach used at present, we propose that
it would be better to try and reduce a few specific problems of public
ill health rather than the present utopian attempt to improve all aspects
of the public's health. Trying to encourage people to lose weight, stop
smoking, take more exercise and eat less saturated fat may well be too
much at once. Too extensive a confrontation results almost inevitably

in frustration for the health educator, and bewilderment for the individual.

It is our opinion that, for the next five years, health education at both national and local level should focus on cigarette smoking. The association between smoking and disease is certain and there is massive evidence that many people wish to stop smoking but need specialised help to do so. Cigarette smoking has already declined in Britain; between 1973 and 1977 the sale of cigarettes fell by 13.6 per cent by weight. Although direct health education has had some success in influencing people, this encouraging decrease probably owes more to indirect health education. In addition, the activities of the pressure group ASH (Action on Smoking and Health) has led to successive price increases. This success indicates among other things, that it is necessary to try to eradicate specific problems. A model of such single-objective education campaigns is described by the International Union against Cancer in their publication 'Lung Cancer Prevention' (UICC 1977).

Too much health education is focused on the group instead of on the individual. Very little is known about what individuals want and too little effort is being devoted to finding out. Most people want freedom from pain and disability. Longevity has only limited appeal, but the nearer death approaches, the greater is the appeal of its postponement. Young people of 15 years of age are not moved to action by the offer of more years of life after 60, but the 59 year old man views his way of life differently if told he is at risk. People wish for freedom from premature death but the definition of 'premature' is much more difficult and subjective than the definition of pain and disability. People wish for freedom from worry and anxiety and they also wish to be free from the intervention of experts and of the state. A final freedom, freedom from boredom, is also essential if people are to be motivated to change.

The Government's White Paper on Prevention and Health was technically sound but ethically weak (HMSO 1977b). Only one of the 83 pages was devoted to the 'Liberty of the individual'. The confident statement is made that 'The real question is not whether the Government should intervene but when and how.' This seems an unwarranted assumption on the part of authority. The true spirit of education embodies the concept of partnership and, when educating for health, individual freedoms no less than any other aspect of personal development must be respected. If health is 'not merely the absence of disease and infirmity' then the liberty of the individual is not merely liberty from illness.

Health education is at present seen as a response to the threat of illness — an afterthought to an educational system which has excluded health. Perhaps the true aim of health education should be to wish for its own extinction, promoting educational and political change towards a society in which health is implicit in every activity.

Acknowledgements

We are grateful for the comments of the editors which led to the article taking its present form. We remain, however, responsible for its contents.

6 HEALTH COSTS OF LIFE STYLE

Margaret Miers

It has become commonplace to note that the orientation of the NHS remains curative, and that concern with the 'environmental' impact on disease has correspondingly been neglected. This paper seeks to redress the balance a little, by exploring the nature of the environmental impact, looking at some groups which are identified as 'at risk'. A significant element in the 'environment' alongside climate or housing is, of course, the social arrangements, customs and habits of any group of people. Life styles are often distinctive, and have distinctive implications for health and disease.

This paper aims to illuminate the importance of life style in helping or hindering the pursuit of health. The relationship between health and life style may be quite complex, but a consideration of mortality and morbidity rates can illustrate it in a sufficiently satisfactory way. Three varieties and aspects of living are examined, leisure patterns of the young, marital relationships, and 'pleasure habits'. The consequences for health of teenagers' 'dare-devil' driving or of enjoying too many cigarettes are fairly often repeated. But that life style carries risks to health and persists into social arrangements far less likely to be considered in this light. Marriage — and the family — is an institution considered by many to be crucial to the structure of our society. Yet even here, there are health costs. Each of the three examples of life styles are considered in turn, and in each the emphasis is on the role and strength of social arrangements and conventions that constrain people to behave in a way that is risky for their health. For, it is argued, it is only by recognising the part played by social factors that a National *Health* Service that lives up to its name can be developed.

Health Costs of Youth Subcultures

In 1975, accidents, particularly motor vehicle accidents, were the most common causes of death for the age group 15-24, an age group with an otherwise low overall mortality rate. Road accident death-rates were higher in this age group than in any other group apart from those over 65.

This high accident rate for young people is not a recent phenomenon. Accidents have been the major cause of death in this age group since the war, with death-rates from motor vehicle traffic accidents rising from 290 per million (males) and 41 per million (females) in 1956 to 362 and 79 per million in 1975. Yet for the same period, increases in death-rates for other age groups are small (OPCS 1975). Furthermore, *casualty* rates from all accidents, whether serious or slight, reflect the sex and age patterns revealed by the death-rates (OPCS 1974).

Two obvious possible explanations of the youthful tendency towards serious and fatal road accidents need some discussion. First, the difference in accident rates for different age groups may be explained by differences in rates of road usage. Young people between 15 and 24 years may use motor vehicles more frequently than their elders. Second, the high accident rates for young people could simply be accounted for by inexperience.

The first of these explanations is relatively easy to discredit. The National Travel Survey carried out by the Department of the Environment in 1972-73 (DoE 1975) indicates that youngsters in their late teens make fewer journeys by car than other age groups apart from persons under 16 or over 60. Furthermore, usage rates for the 30-59 age group are similar to rates for the 21-29 age group, yet these similar usage rates result in markedly discrepant rates of injury. Thus differences in road use seem an unlikely explanation for age differences in numbers of accidents. However, the sex differences in accident rates may be partially accounted for by rates of use. In all age groups, women's accident death-rates are low compared with men's and women also make fewer journeys by car than men.

The second explanation cannot be discounted. Details of driving experience invariably support the view that youthful accident rates are at least partly a product of inexperience on the roads. In 1972/73, of all those with a full driver's licence, only 24 per cent were under 30 and of those with a full licence for six years or more, only 14 per cent were in the under-thirty age group (National Travel Survey). Thus, with young drivers, the effects of age and inexperience can easily be confused. Despite research in a variety of settings, this confusion remains to be disentangled. A study of motor coach drivers revealed experience to be more important as there was no association between age and accidents when experience was held constant (Brown and Ghiselli 1948). However, in studies of industrial accidents, researchers have found that, whilst experience was the most critical variable in the initial year of service, age also played some part since the initial accident rate of younger workers was significantly higher than that of workers in older age groups (Adelstein 1952; van Zelst 1954). These varied and conflicting findings can only suggest that age remains as a possible significant factor in accident causation.

A great many characteristics of youth have been suggested as reasons for youthful accident proneness: bravado, chance-taking, drinking, lack of judgement, peer group pressure toward irresponsible behaviour, inexperience, inattention, indiscipline, impulsiveness, recklessness, overestimation of capacity, pride, lack of family responsibilities, producing a lack of care. Few of these factors, however, have ever been empirically investigated. The exception is drinking. Much research has demonstrated the deleterious effect of drinking on driving skills and the relationship between alcohol consumption and road accidents. In addition, drinking is a growing problem among the young. Yet alcohol appears to be a factor in only a low proportion of young persons' accidents. One survey shows that the highest accident rate *without* alcoholic involvement occurred at ages 18-20 (Pelz *et al.* 1975). Thus alcohol plays no part in many of the accidents which involve young people.

Despite the importance of acquiring a job to achieve 'manhood', having a job of work to do may do little for the adolescent's sense of purpose and identity. The opportunities for interesting jobs are very limited, frustrating initiative, aptitude and energy. If daily life fails to provide a young person with the chance to show skill or initiative, or to gain a sense of achievement, such opportunities must and will be created. This will happen even though the chosen activities are not only useless to the society, but destructive to the well-being of the participants themselves.

Some of the other factors, such as lack of judgement and overestimation of capability, could be related to inexperience at performing specific skills. Yet misjudgement is also associated with bravado and chance-taking, behaviour often encouraged in youth peer groups. The presence of such characteristics among young people may be explained by their shared problems arising from their quest for a valued social status and identity.

The social position of young people in contemporary society is an ambiguous one, with a confusing mix of expectations and obligations. They are between childhood and adulthood for long periods. Physically mature at an early age they are denied the opportunity to achieve the status of a working adult by the prolonged period of education and training which is seen as necessary for the development of the complex and demanding skills of adulthood in the modern industrialised world. The problem for adolescents, then, is one of personal adjustments to a period where their social status and social role are not clearly defined. The search for a personal, and adult, identity can lead to excessive indulgence in what appears to be 'adult' forms of behaviour – smoking, drinking, driving – or to the development of norms of behaviour which are deliberately 'anti-adult'. Lacking financial or family responsibilities, young people can make a virtue out of irresponsibility; lacking a meaningful job to do, doing nothing or investing energy in purely leisure pursuits becomes a positive aim, bringing its own excitement.

The development of youth movements is not a recent phenomenon but one that has been accentuated by various post-war changes in Britain. The school-leaving age has steadily increased as have opportunities for further and higher education. Hence many youngsters have experienced a forced extension of the period for 'becoming an adult'. An increase in leisure time for all workers, and of course for young people denied the opportunity to work, coupled with the increased affluence both of teenagers (Abrams 1959) and of their parents during post-war years led to the development of 'youth oriented' leisure industries which exploited the potential of youth as a mass market. In addition post-war Britain became a society which relied on mass communications for its knowledge and news. Thus TV and magazines brought the means of mass manipulation and imitation into the homes of every family. Distinctive styles of dress for teenagers served the needs of both the young people themselves and the needs of a growing economy. As Hall and Jefferson have commented 'Youth, compared to age, were direct beneficiaries of the welfare state and educational opportunities, least constrained by older patterns of and attitudes to, spending or consumption; most involved in a guilt free commitment to pleasure and immediate satisfactions' (Hall and Jefferson 1975). It is hardly surprising if the older generation found such involvement morally reprehensible, in view of their own youthful experiences during the war and the Depression. Equally, though, the responses of contemporary youth must be understood within the context of the society in which they live.

From the above comments it is easy to think that it is possible to identify a distinctive hedonistic and rebellious life style which warrants the label 'youth culture'. Indeed, many writers have developed this image of cultural differences in contemporary Britain. But it is important to make two major points which limit the usefulness of the concept of 'youth culture'. First, many aspects of behaviour associated with young people – rebellion, bravado, chance-taking, violence and delinquency – are, in fact, mainly characteristics of male, not female, youth.

Young women appear to indulge in rebellious behaviour less frequently than men. This may be because women have been largely ignored in research into youth subcultures or because women do not have problems whilst adolescents and hence are not forced to create deviant solutions. Goodman's view is that women are not expected to be useful in society; they are expected to occupy a crucial role only in the family structure and provided this role is attainable, young girls find adolescence comparatively easy (Goodman 1961). Indeed, if it is the case that girls' aspirations are mainly confined to marriage and motherhood, they are more successful now than before the war, in that the average age of marriage is lower and children are borne earlier, though in fewer numbers. Furthermore, women marry earlier than men. Hence for many girls, marrying shortly after completing full-time education, self-fulfilment and a satisfactory social role, with attendant responsibility, may well seem close at hand.

The role of young women, and their aspirations, raises the second important point in relation to 'youth culture', that of the relationship between the life style of youth and the dominant culture. Youthful behaviour may differ from that of the older generation but many of the focal concerns and the accepted patterns of behaviour remain closely linked to those of the dominant culture. Hence in youth groups, as in the wider community, women play a subordinate and often submissive role. The adolescent world reflects as well as rebels against the adult world; it constitutes not an independent culture, but a subculture.

This is clearly illustrated by returning to the discussion of car use and road traffic accidents among teenagers. The motor car is far more than a means of transportation; to the nation it is an index of economic prosperity, to citizens it may be a symbol of status, to some minorities it can be a sign of equality, and for many it is a symbol of wealth and prestige. Small wonder, then, that the car, a symbol of the affluent consumer society, should become an important sign of maturity, independence, financial success and status for many of the youth of that society. Youthful values stem from the parent culture.

For young people the car has specific utility — it gives its user freedom and mobility, provides the opportunity for romantic conquest and allows for the easy pursuit of leisure activities. People aged 21-29 are in the age group most likely to use a car for social and personal visits (National Travel Survey 1975). But cars are also part of the search for a satisfactory public identity and they can be chosen, decorated and displayed for their status rather than their use value. Perhaps more significantly, the car is also a symbol of power. It encourages speed, daring and excitement. Indeed society respects and rewards those drivers who court danger, albeit on the racing track. Such drivers are sportsmen who espouse the necessary values of competitiveness and courage. Again, then, it is hardly surprising that the young male may use the road to show off his developing masculinity by fast driving, by taking chances, by showing his courage, his decisiveness and hopefully his skill. Adults may disapprove, but, if we are to believe the advertisements, his friends, and of course his girlfriends, will be impressed. In a society where risk-taking can be seen as an economic virtue it is not surprising that youngsters attempting to maintain a shaky foothold in adulthood will take the greatest risks. In taking chances in order to find independence, freedom, power and confidence, the young man is not only a victim of his own folly and of his peers' life style, but of the dominant societal values, and stereotypes of masculinity.

Mental Health Costs of Marriage

It is not only the relationship between youthfulness and health costs that is worthy of careful investigation. Significant differences in mortality and morbidity rates are also apparent between men and women. Men have higher death-rates than women, but women report symptoms of both physical and mental illness more frequently, and women utilise physician and hospital services for these conditions at higher rates than men (Nathanson 1975). The difference between rates of illness for men and for women is particularly marked in relation to mental illness (Gove and Tudor 1973).

The reasons for the discrepancies between men and women's rates of mortality and morbidity, and the differences in their susceptibility to mental illness, appear to be socio-cultural rather than physiological (Waldron 1976). It is men's life style which produces health costs resulting in different death-rates. So women's life style may help cause high rates of physical and mental morbidity, though relationships between behaviour and morbidity are not clear. Some clues to the relationships lie in differences in rates of mortality and morbidity according to marital status. For both men and women the married have lower mortality rates than the single, widowed and divorced. However, the differences are much greater for men than for women. Morbidity rates reveal a slightly different pattern. Women, but not men, have lower general morbidity rates when married, but married women have higher rates of depressive illness than the single, widowed and divorced (General Household Survey, OPCS 1975; Porter 1970). Indeed marriage appears to be a status that induces psychological well-being in men, hence providing protection from physical illness too. Gove (1973) has argued that the differences in mortality rates according to marital status are largely due to specific types of mortality such as suicide, homicide, accidents, lung cancer, cirrhosis of the liver, diabetes and TB, all conditions where an individual's psychological state may affect life chances.

Whereas marriage appears to protect men from stresses and strains, it appears to produce stresses for women. The marked differences in rates of mental illness for men and women apply only for the married populations. Gove and Tudor (1973), in an extensive review of the evidence, found that since the Second World War married women have higher rates of mental ill health than married men, but single, widowed and divorced males are more likely to suffer from mental illness than single, widowed and divorced females. Married women's susceptibility to mental illness appears to be a relatively recent phenomenon. Prior to World War II many studies indicated higher rates of mental illness for men than for women. It appears then that it is nót the general expectations of the feminine role that induce symptoms, but the expectations and obligations of marriage which produce psychological disturbance in women. Support for this argument lies in the fact that mental health is better amongst divorced and widowed women — the formerly married — than it is among married women.

Gove and Tudor (1973) pinpoint a number of factors which they see as characteristic of the married woman's role in contemporary society. Married women are often restricted to one major activity, that of housewifery, which is unstructured and frustrating, restricting and boring. This may lead to much time to brood over troubles, develop and notice symptoms, and adopt the sick role. Even when in work a married woman may find herself frustrated as married women are frequently employed in occupational positions not commensurate with their educational background. When working the married woman will experience the strains of performing the multiple roles of housewife, mother and breadwinner, which may lead to role conflict, stress, tension and signs of mental illness. In addition all married women are subjected to conflicting and confusing social expectations which lead to problems in identifying priorities and achieving personal satisfaction. Gove and Tudor suggest that the diffuse expectations of adult women are a result of recent changes in women's role; the increased emancipation of women has forced them to bear the mental costs of a diversified life style.

Ann Oakley (1974a) has argued that there are certain features of housework which create dissatisfaction and frustration. First and foremost, the housewife is isolated from social contacts and spends much of her time alone in her own home. In Oakley's study of housewives loneliness was a frequent complaint. Housework, though made up of a number of different tasks, is also monotonous and fragmented and is often seen as of low status and trivial. In addition, the housewife has a long working week. Unsurprisingly, 70 per cent of Oakley's sample of housewives were dissatisfied with the job of housework. Oakley argues that it is intrinsic features of housework and the conditions under which it is done that act as dissatisfiers. A woman's own domesticity, educational background, and social class grouping, may be much less important as variables influencing housework satisfaction/dissatisfaction than is usually thought.

Housewives may develop techniques of routinisation and specification of standards in order to overcome the monotonous, fragmented nature of the tasks, and to award themselves some psychological rewards for achieving goals. Thus housewives can cope with the difficulties of carrying out unstructured and unsupervised tasks, but at the same time pursuit of reward and satisfaction can lead to obsessionalism and excessive housepride. Such behaviour often appears neurotic, though it may be an inevitable outcome of an enforced life style. Hence it appears that the limited nature of the housewife's role may induce mental health costs.

An alternative view however is that role conflict and role strain causes mental illness in married women. As Gove and Tudor argue, women are expected to be breadwinners, mother and housewife. Although plausible, this explanation finds little empirical support. In general it appears that employment outside the home protects women from symptoms of mental illness, even in marriage (Nathanson 1975). Furthermore confinement to the home increases the likelihood of male dissatisfaction and depression. Gove (1973) found that some studies of mental illness rates show that the rates of married men and women are similar after retirement, when both marriage partners lack occupational status. A further American study (US Dept. HEW 1970), comparing psychological stress symptom rates between housewives and unemployed men, found similar high rates in the two groups. Certainly men may feel the lack of job status more acutely than women, given the differences in the societal expectations of their role, but these findings do suggest that it may be the life style of a housebound wife that encourages neuroses and depression.

Many women, of course, are confined to the home and to housewifery, because of young children. Although women may find aspects of child care intrinsically satisfying, the presence of young children increases their immobility, isolation and household chores. Research indicates that although motherhood may prevent women from perceiving physical symptoms, it does not appear to protect them from the housewife's depression, dissatisfaction and neuroses (Nathanson 1975; Oakley 1974a).

Many commentators have recently argued, however, that the married roles of women are undergoing change. The increase in numbers of married women working has led to the suggestion that the married roles of men and women will become 'symmetrical' (Young and Willmott 1973), with both partners working outside the home and sharing the tasks of breadwinner, houseperson and parent. There is reason to doubt, as Oakley (1974a) does, that there is in fact any significant change taking place in the roles of husband and wife, despite women's movement into the workforce. The evidence for a move towards domestic equality stems from a limited series of questions about household and child-care tasks, generally showing that men do help with the washing up and play with their offspring. Such participation in domestic chores, however, though greater now than before the war, does not mean that men and women share these chores equally. Oakley (1974a) found that only 15 per cent of husbands had a high level of participation in housework and 25 per cent a high level of participation in child care. From this she concludes that 'only a minority of husbands give the kind of help that assertions of equality in modern marriage imply' (Oakley 1974a: 138). Whatever the future may bring, at present it seems unlikely that male participation in home life alleviates the burden of housewifery from married women to any significant extent. Women rarely enjoy an equal division of labour within the home.

A second characteristic of the supposedly developing equal and symmetrical family is an increase in the companionship of husband and wife. The modern married couple are seen as developing 'joint' conjugal roles (cf. Bott 1971) where activities inside and outside the home are shared. Yet much research casts doubt on the 'companionship' of modern marriage particularly among semi- and unskilled families. Komarovsky, in a study of American family life (Komarovsky 1967) presents a vivid picture of poor communication in marriage, with men failing to discuss their job satisfactions and dissatisfactions with their wives and women unable to talk to their husbands about personal worries about health, personal aspirations and dissatisfactions. It is likely that role-segregated marriages remain more common than commentators would wish them to be.

Oakley (1976:100) considers that

> this pattern of marital roles, though one in which both man and woman suffer from a paucity of communication, is a situation that holds particular stresses for women. It continually reinforces their traditional identification with domesticity in a society that has reduced and devalued the rewards domesticity has to offer. The widening of opportunities for women outside the home which has occurred in recent decades has had very little impact on the lives of the majority of women, who are brought up to believe in marriage as a woman's life-goal and who then find themselves restricted by marriage — by the segregation between husband and wife roles which marriage entails — to the sphere of domestic interests.

Thus it must be women's continued entrapment, for a time at least, in the frustrations of a housewife's life style that largely accounts for the prevalence of neuroses and depression among married women. It it is indeed the case that the future marital relationship will become one of equality and companionship, then we can look forward to an improvement in the mental health of women. But if the symmetrical family remains a dream and not reality, we can expect not only continued increases in divorce rates but growing numbers of neurotic and depressed women. The mental health costs of marriage will remain.

Health Costs of Pleasure Habits

In addition to sex differences in rates of mental illness, it is well known that there are also class differences (Holingshead and Redlich 1958). Indeed there is a class gradient in mortality rates for men and women, in rates of consulting general practitioners, attending outpatient departments, absenteeism from work for health reasons, and other measures of morbidity. There are many reasons for such differences, ranging from the nature of the job, living conditions, diet, to personal habits, attitudes and beliefs. One particular pleasure habit, smoking, could alone account for many of the discrepancies. Mortality from lung cancer and from bronchitis, for example, show particularly marked class gradients, with the higher social classes having the lower rates. These two diseases are associated with cigarette smoking. Cigarette smoking is more common among manual than non-manual workers. Manual workers spend a higher proportion of their household income on tobacco than other groups, and have higher rates of cigarette consumption (OPCS 1975). Furthermore, as a group, they are the slowest to change. Over the past decade there have been quite substantial reductions in the proportions of smokers in the population, and, for the first time, household expenditure on tobacco decreased in 1977. But these changes are not uniformly distributed throughout the population; it is the top social classes who are altering their behaviour; social classes IV and V, the semi- and unskilled workers, are reluctant to give up. Smoking remains the norm rather than the exception. Unavoidably their health suffers.

The fact that individuals persist with pleasure habits which damage their health, despite repeated warnings, is a major problem for practitioners and policy makers in the NHS. The problem is that in order to stop smoking people first have to recognise that they are 'at risk' if they continue. People who feel healthy may find it difficult to accept that they risk becoming ill later. To stop smoking in order to avoid future risk involves depriving themselves in the present. Not only are they obliged to alter their behaviour for no immediate rewards but the future gain is negative and impossible to identify. We are encouraged to cease smoking in order to avoid ill health in the future and bad breath and smelly clothes in the present, but there are few immediate rewards to be gained as even the financial advantage is cumulative rather than instantaneous and, for many people, giving up smoking will not even guarantee social approval. On the contrary it may bring ridicule and social unease. It receives little support from other people. Giving up involves individuals in calculating statistical probabilities about forms of behaviour and health threats, in taking responsibility for one's own actions and in acting now and for an indefinite period in order to ensure a possible pay-off at some unknown and unknowable date. Unsurprisingly this orientation towards the future, the belief that the future may be controlled, and the emphasis placed on individual effort and delayed gratification does not fit in with everyone's life style and attitudes towards the world.

The clue to the reasons why professional and managerial workers — 'the middle class' — have given up smoking more readily than the manual workers — 'the working class' — lies in their general life experience, life style and social norms rather than their particular views about smoking. Differences between the attitudes and aspirations of different social classes have been well documented. Goldthorpe and Lockwood (1969) have identified three ways in which manual and non-manual workers differ in their behaviour and thinking. First, middle and working class differ in their views about the determinants of social circumstances, about the nature of society and about the purpose of life. In the traditional working-class perspective, society is divided into 'us' and 'them' and the division between the two groups is unbridgeable. For the individual, his social circumstances are 'given', facts of life, which have to be accepted and 'put up with'. In contrast, in the middle-class perspective, society is hierarchically organised and it is possible to move up and down the different strata according to one's individual effort or lack of it. The future, and man's place in society, is his own responsibility and it is his duty to 'make the most of himself' and to try to 'get on'.

A second major difference between middle- and working-class perspectives is that the working class, making the best out of life as it is, live in, and for, the present, whilst the middle class, intent on 'getting on', attach importance to looking and planning ahead. The manual worker is a 'short-term hedonist'; the professional worker or manager favours 'deferred gratification'.

A final important difference between the attitudes in the two social groups is the emphasis placed on the importance of individual or group effort. Manual workers stress the importance of collective action for achieving goals; the middle-class workers value individual effort as the main mode of achieving change.

Goldthorpe and Lockwood's discussion of the two perspectives involves exaggeration and oversimplifications, but there is substantial research evidence to support their argument, both from their own and other studies of middle- and working-class attitudes and behaviour (Hoggart 1958; Komarovsky 1967; J. and E. Newson 1970; Bott 1971). Furthermore the perspectives of each class are not unrealistic, stemming almost inevitably from their different social environments. A non-manual worker, earning a monthly salary, is forced to plan for a few weeks ahead, thus encouraging a future-oriented outlook. Such an outlook is reinforced by the career structure and long-term benefits such as increments and pensions which are associated with middle-class jobs. The manual weekly wage earner lives to a different time scale. 'Wage packets come in weekly and go out weekly' (Hoggart 1958:133). Manual workers suffer from comparatively high rates of unemployment and their chances of rising to a higher status occupation and gaining more financial rewards are comparatively slight (Harris and Clausen 1966). Thus the worker whose daily life and job is insecure, sees the future as insecure, accepts his fate, and lives for the present. This attitude helps explain patterns of working-class expenditure. Once immediate dues are paid, much of the remaining money is spent on extravagances. The working-class view is that 'pleasures are a central part of life, not something perhaps to be allowed after a great number of other commitments have been met' (Hoggart 1958:134). Money alone will not bring security, so excess money will be spent. Friends, family, and the local community – not money – bring security to working-class men and women. They are not swayed by abstract arguments but are persuaded by direct, personal contacts. Their interest in and dependency on other people develops naturally from their traditional modes of living, in densely populated terraced streets, and their proximity at work, on the factory floor. The middle class, however, in more spacious suburban houses, with more formal education and more opportunities to exercise individual responsibility at work, find it easier and more natural to rely on individual decisions and on self-help.

The constraints of the 'at-risk role', therefore, are more acceptable to the middle class and it is unsurprising that it is they who are ready to take action to preserve their health. Calculating future health costs is congruent with middle-class orientations, but to give up the smoking habit without immediate benefit would contradict the working-class values on 'short-term hedonism'. Smoking cigarettes is one of the working-class pleasures which are a 'central part of life'. This reluctance to take preventive action despite knowledge of health risks is not confined to the smoking habit. Working-class women, for example, are less likely than middle-class women to have a cervical smear test (Wakefield and Sansom 1966), and more likely to report unintentional pregnancies (Cartwright 1970, Rainwater 1960). Rainwater argues that the lack of contraceptive use among manual couples in his survey was due, at least in part, to a fatalistic, present orientation. This fatalism and present orientation, together with the importance of pleasure pursuits, helps to account for working-class reluctance to give up smoking.

Thus the National Health Service faces the problem of a drain on resources through self-induced health costs which derive, at least partly, from the smoking habit. It also faces the challenge of persuading individuals of all classes to give up smoking for the sake of their health, and of devising policies which will enable anti-smoking feeling to flourish. How does the NHS rise to this challenge?

At the policy level, the government faces the problem that, whilst wishing to adopt a critical and concerned policy towards smoking, cigarettes provide a major source of revenue. Britain has been slow to impose restrictions on smoking in public places compared with some other countries, and government finance for anti-smoking education remains paltry. In March 1977 £1 million were given to the Health Education Council to put over the anti-smoking message, but a couple of months later £8 million were spent by tobacco companies on competitive brand advertising to promote tobacco substitute cigarettes.

Various professional groups within the National Health Service are, of course, concerned with educating the public about smoking risks. General practitioners and health visitors seem particularly well placed to carry out this work. The GPs' potential as health educators lies in their unique opportunity for persuasion whilst seeing patients in their daily work, and in their special authority and status in the eyes of the public. However, research into patterns of behaviour change indicates that the public do not perceive general practitioners as an important source of influence, and there is no evidence to suggest that GPs are effective in altering smoking behaviour (Bluck 1975). Perhaps because of their training, GPs' attitudes towards preventive medicine are often ambiguous and their participation in health education limited (Bluck 1975, Section V).

Health visitors, however, have health education as one of their main aims, but it is difficult to find evidence concerning their role in encouraging changes in smoking behaviour. Successful communication about future health risks between middle-class professionals and working-class clients seems unlikely in view of the class differences in attitudes and life style already discussed. Mayer and Timms's (1969) study of social work points out that much of the failure of social workers to help clients stemmed from a fundamental lack of understanding of each other because of their different approaches to problem solving. For a middle-class doctor or health visitor, belief in the importance and possibility of individual control over one's own decisions and future, and responsibility for one's own behaviour and own health, and a facility for abstract argument, may lead to a mode of communication which is insufficiently personal and directive for a patient who is looking for immediate and specific advice. There is a danger that both professional and client will not realise that his own values are not shared values.

The health visitor, in particular, may encounter these dangers. Her major task is to promote the healthy development of young children, thus working closely with mothers and families. Health visitors can, therefore, be at the front line of the care and prevention of depression and neuroses among married women. An understanding of the nature and consequences of contemporary family relationships should enable the health visitor to identify some of the reasons for the mental health costs of marriage. Yet in much sociology, social commentary, and health visitor training, the view of the family is a glorified one, indirectly seeking to uphold a sentimental or ideal model of family relationships. Indeed writers and teachers about the family may themselves live under the unusual conditions of relative symmetry in their role relationships and consequently be insensitive to differences between their own, and others', family experiences. Health visitors in particular need to develop their critical faculties concerning the family in order to cope with the daily problems which, through their clients, they are forced to face. As Oakley (1976:101) has commented, 'a critical approach to the family need not be either destructive or pessimistic. Its proper concern is simply the avoidance of false diagnosis and treatment based on erroneous premises. A plea for the reconsideration of conventional explanations and treatments is a plea for the discernment of the social causes of illness, where these exist. In the case of the family and marriage, sentiment probably gets in the way of science more than most of us realise.'

Sentiment also gets in the way of discussion about problems of youth. Young people are seen as espousing the worthless values of hedonism and spontaneity instead of the traditional values of hard work and discipline. The young are seen as a problem to society rather than as a problem to themselves. Thus the serious health costs through accidents which youthfulness can inflict are rarely discussed and analysed. Yet high accident rates among young people, like mental illness among married women and lung cancer deaths among the working class, are inevitable consequences of the life styles of these social groups. In competitive, industrialised societies, different social groups enjoy different social positions and privileges. Those successful in the world of work can enjoy the rewards which the society can bestow, including a long and healthy life and relative freedom from health costs. Social groups which lack economic power and social status incur certain health costs which derive from the constraints on their life style imposed directly or indirectly by their low position in the economic hierarchy. Thus young men, seeking an adult identity and status, suffer from their own recklessness; married women, constrained by their 'non-productive' role of housewife, suffer from isolation and boredom, and semi- and unskilled manual workers, lacking long-term financial security, gratify themselves by immediate pleasures which impose health risks.

These health costs of life style demonstrate the importance of considering the effects of the social environment on an individual's psychology and biology. They pinpoint the need for the philosophy of the National Health Service to be a service concerned not just with the physiological components of a person, but also with personal relationships, attitudes and values, hopes and aspirations, and the 'whole' person at home, at work and in the wider social environment.

Acknowledgements

I should like to thank Anne Murcott for her help and support in the preparation of this paper.

7 THE NATIONAL HEALTH SERVICE AND ITS RELEVANCE TO INDUSTRIAL HEALTH AND SAFETY

Denis Gregory

Introduction

From the establishment and report of the Robens Committee (Department of Employment 1972) to the setting up of the Health and Safety Commission (HSC) and Health and Safety Executive (HSE), the past decade has witnessed a steadily growing concern for the health and safety of individuals at work. This concern has expressed itself primarily in calls for tougher controls over hazards at work, more stringent enforcement policies, more extensive obligations on employers to cater for the safety and welfare of their employees and greater involvement of the workforce itself in the regulation of safety. To an extent, the passage and subsequent refinement of the Health and Safety at Work Act 1974 has provided a response to these calls.

In contrast, over the same period, very little pressure has been brought to bear on the need to improve our occupational health service provision. The Employment Medical Advisory Service Act 1972 (subsequently replaced by similar provisions within the Health and Safety at Work Act 1974) established a greater government commitment to independent medical *advice* to industry, and more recently the HSC's discussion document on occupational health services has attempted to provoke some form of debate (Health and Safety Commission 1977). Yet the central provision of such a service has remained curiously free from any widespread and effective criticism.

Apart from the nationalised industries, where a commitment to occupational health service provision is part of their founding Acts, there are no statutory requirements placed upon private industry, other than references to the provision of first aid facilities in the Factories Act 1961. In the absence of a centralised occupational health service it has been left to industry to develop its own provision voluntarily. However, as a recent EMAS survey (quoted in Health and Safety Commission 1977) has shown, those services that do exist are patchy in coverage and variable in the quality and quantity of resources devoted to them. Although the more obvious (i.e. long-established) hazards of industry seem to be becoming less of a problem as employers have been forced to provide improved controls and more effective engineering solutions, their place has been taken by a whole host of far more insidious technological and toxic hazards which are equally, if not more, threatening to the well-being of the workforce.

The rest of this chapter sets out to examine the current state of occupational health service provision, the need for more comprehensive cover and the possible future role of the NHS. We begin with a brief review of the historical development of occupational health service provision and with an examination of the post-war debate as to the desirability of an occupational health service being provided as part of the NHS.

The Development of Occupational Health Services

The following comment is to be found in the Health and Safety Commission's recent discussion document on occupational health services:

> Concern to protect the workers from occupational disease does not appear to have been the main motive force behind the historical development of occupational health services in this country.

The 'motive' forces were supplied by the Factory Act of 1844 which required the appointment of 'Certifying Factory Surgeons' whose sole function was to ensure that children were old enough to enter employment. The 1855 Factory Act extended this function to include a requirement to certify that young people were not incapacitated for work by disease or bodily infirmity. Factory surgeons were also to be allowed to investigate industrial accidents. The Workman's Compensation Act of 1897 led employers to appoint physicians to protect themselves (rather than their workers) against claims for compensation. It is true that there were a few enlightened employers in the eighteenth and nineteenth centuries who provided general medical and nursing care to their employees, and pioneering physicians such as Rott, who showed the relationship between soot and scrotal cancer in chimney sweeps in 1775, and Thackrah, who published his more comprehensive work on occupational diseases in 1832. But parliamentary, industrial and medical involvement in the fostering of occupational health services up until the foundation of the 'Welfare State' remained piecemeal and less than constructive.

The post-war period from the 'birth' of the Welfare State to the present day has been marked by indecision and conflicting advice from a variety of bodies, both governmental and otherwise. The Gower Committee in 1949 recognised the need for occupational health services for non-industrial employment (Committee of Enquiry into Health, Safety and Welfare in Non-Industrial Employment 1949). Shortly afterwards in 1951 the Dale Committee, set up by the government specifically to examine industrial medical services, concluded that such services should be encouraged and did not duplicate NHS facilities (Committee of Enquiry on Industrial Health Services 1951). In contrast, the Robens Committee, some 20 years later, took a more or less opposite view which stressed the danger of wasteful duplication of the NHS. This latter view was formed despite the opinions of both the forerunner of the CBI, which had urged its member firms to provide occupational health facilities in order to minimise the loss of working time, and the Alexander Committee (British Medical Association 1961). This committee, formed by the British Medical Association, advocated greater government involvement in the provision of occupational health services for those firms which did not already have them.

The trade union position is more consistent and provides us with a sharper focus on the failings of existing provision and the possibilities for improvement within the NHS. The 1944 Annual Congress passed a resolution calling for:

> the Government to provide an Industrial Medical Service within the projected NHS on a basis which will ensure that –
> a) all medical personnel shall be responsible only to the Service and the State
> b) the Industrial Medical Service shall become operative in all sections of industry and commerce.

As a result of this clear and unequivocal call two delegations from the General Council of the TUC had meetings in 1945 with the then Ministers of Health and Labour. In response to the TUC's insistence that the proposed NHS should embrace an industrial medical service the Minister of Health, whilst expressing sympathy, argued that there was insufficient parliamentary time to deal with a complete integration of the health service. Ernest Bevin, then Minister of Labour, addressing himself to the first part of the 1944 Resolution, made, according to the TUC Annual Report of 1945 (p. 73), the following remarks:

> he used to believe that a factory Doctor should be a state employee, but now he felt that the employer should pay for the medical service

and that it should be part of the managerial responsibility.

The 1944 resolution has pretty well remained the basis on which all subsequent representations to the government have been made. It has, however, been refined by a resolution passed at the Annual Congress in 1968 and a detailed memorandum issued by the General Council in 1969. In this the General Council made the important distinction that a comprehensive occupational health service should be geared to deal with the effects of work on health and the effects of health on work.

The TUC stressed that the former function must include the 'recognition, evaluation and control' of all occupational hazards whether 'physical, chemical, biological or psychosocial' and emphasised that occupational health personnel would be expected to carry out environmental and clinical observation to evaluate effects of exposure to hazards at the workplace. The clear inference made here by the TUC is that an occupational health service should have functions extending well beyond the mere treatment of accident and disease victims, to an active involvement in the process and system of accident and disease prevention.

By 1969 there was a degree of consensus between the TUC, the forerunner of the CBI and the BMA on the concept of, and need for, an expanded occupational health provision. Yet despite 30 years of committees and consistent trade union pressure, despite the development of occupational health services in the nationalised sector and for government employees, successive governments have refused to give even a commitment to the incorporation of an occupational health service within the NHS.

Current Occupational Health Service Provision

Apart from the early arguments over the possibilities of wasteful duplication of resources, it has been contended by successive governments that existing voluntary occupational health services allied to local NHS facilities are sufficient to cope with likely demand. This, of course, assumes that voluntary occupational health services either are, or will become, reasonably widespread in terms of their coverage and efficiency as far as the working population is concerned. It also assumes that suitable NHS facilities will remain readily accessible to those needing treatment for injuries or diseases suffered at work. In the event, little evidence can be shown which supports the former of these assumptions and some doubt must persist over the latter.

A survey, carried out in 1976 for the Employment Medical Advisory Service, using a sample of 3,000 manufacturing and construction companies in the private sector, showed that 85 per cent of the firms surveyed employing some 34 per cent of the sample workforce provided no occupational health service other than first aiders employed less than ten hours a week in that capacity. Over and above this, only 0.5 per cent of the companies employing 16.5 per cent of the workforce provided full-time medical and nursing staff. Some 47 per cent of the workforce were covered by various combinations of part-time medical and other nursing staff.

There are as yet no indications or evaluations of the effectiveness of voluntary occupational health provision within the various subsectors of private manufacturing industry. We can, however, form a crude picture of those sub sectors which would seem to be most in need of some form of occupational health provision. Table 7.1 shows the incidence rates of what are termed 'group 1' accidents, that is serious but not fatal injuries. These are compared on a standard industrial classification basis with the corresponding occupational health provision as revealed by the EMAS survey.

Table 7.1 shows that there is no correspondence between the availability of occupational health care and accident rates. Hence it is not safe to assume that the more obviously dangerous subsectors will have a correspondingly high provision of occupational health services. Moreover, the relatively high level of provision within the nationalised industries will not affect this conclusion greatly since in only three of the sectors shown (coal and petroleum products, metal manufacture and vehicles) can there be said to be any significant degree of nationalisation.

The information provided in Table 7.1 must be regarded, at best, as a rough indication of the 'supply and demand' for occupational health provision in the manufacturing and construction sectors, and it should be remembered that significant numbers of the insured workforce are not included in these data. Nevertheless, manufacturing and construction currently account for around 40 per cent of the working population. Within these sectors slightly more than half of the labour force are distributed amongst firms employing less than 500 workers. Given the clear relationship the EMAS survey found between size of company and extent of occupational health service cover, it can be seen that for these workers the reliance on 'voluntarism' has produced little more than first aid boxes and good intentions.

The doubt over the suggestion that most factories and offices are

Table 7.1: The Frequency of Serious Accidents and the Provision of Occupational Health Services by Industry Sub-Group

Industry (SIC)	Incidence rate of group 1 accidents per 100,000 workers					% of firms with:	
	1972	1973	1974	1975	1976	Medical and/or Nursing Staff	Occ. Health Service of any kind
Food, drink & tobacco	710	800	630	660	690	17.6	39.0
Coal & petrol products	590	1210	770	960	n.a.	33.3	55.5
Chemicals & allied	640	640	710	650	620	25.3	42.8
Metal manuf.	1000	920	1110	970	920	28.0	42.2
Mech. eng.	730	640	730	650	680	9.5	30.0
Inst. eng.	190	270	260	280	n.a.	17.8	34.8
Elect. eng.	350	400	310	290	310	18.7	46.2
Vehicles	470	410	440	420	350	36.0	59.7
Metal goods NCS	740	770	680	740	660	9.2	27.7
Textiles	560	590	440	460	490	12.6	27.1
Clothing & footwear	130	110	120	130	210	4.9	15.1
Bricks, pot, glass & cement	930	850	710	690	890	9.6	32.0
Timber & furniture	950	690	940	660	890	4.0	14.7
Paper, print & publ.	530	530	520	340	530	6.1	21.2
Other manuf.	580	470	440	360	490	11.4	30.0
Construction	820	710	760	740	680	1.9	4.1

Source: Occupational Health Services: The Way Ahead, and HSE 1976 Report on Manufacturing and Service Industries

located within easy reach of existing NHS facilities must be sharpened as more and more peripheral NHS hospitals are either closed or their facilities (particularly casualty departments) cut back, as a result of expenditure restraint and the trend towards the centralisation of hospital resources. Increasingly, this could mean that workers requiring immediate hospital attention may have to face long, painful and possibly fatal, ambulance journeys.

The Need for an Improved Occupational Health Service

The belief that industry has become safer in the post-war period of economic growth is one of our more misguided examples of conventional wisdom (e.g. Ministry of Labour 1956). There are indeed indicators suggesting that industry *should* have become safer. For example, the number of manual workers, who have traditionally been considered to be most 'at risk' whilst working, have declined: the most recent census data show a drop from 55.3 per cent of the economically active population recorded in 1966 to 46.4 per cent in the 1971 Census; currently, the proportion is probably around 40 per cent. Further evidence of this can be seen in the fall in weekly hours worked per operative in manufacturing industry. This has dropped from an index (1962 = 100) of 100.4 in 1958 to 75.1 in 1977. Regrettably, accidents in industry are not declining at the same rate. The somewhat restricted data available from the Factory Inspectorate, i.e. statistics relating to fatalities and reportable accidents in manufacturing and construction industries, show a welcome fall in registered fatalities from 799 in 1930 to 427 in 1975. However, all reportable accidents, that is those causing at least three days' absence from work and including fatalities, have shown a sharp rise from 193,059 in 1950, to a post-war peak of 322,390 in 1969 to the 1975 level of 243, 140.

Various reasons are put forward to explain this latter trend. First it is argued that as both company and state sickness schemes have improved, so the propensity of workers to take three or more days' sick-leave as a result of an accident has also increased. Second, it is said that the Factory Inspectorate has become progressively tougher on the non-reporting of accidents, hence companies are now more efficient in this respect. There is probably some truth in both of these contentions. But neither offers a sufficient explanation for the post-war rise in reportable accidents, given the positive advantages which should have flowed from the changing balance between manual and non-manual workers in the labour force. Moreover, whilst absolute levels of fatalities from accidents have declined, the incidence rates of fatal and non-fatal accidents have remained stable across all sectors of industry. Table 7.2 shows the fatality and total accident incidence rates per 100,000 employees at risk.

Table 7.2: Accident Incidence Rates per 100,000 Workers at Risk: 1971-75[a]

	1971	1972	1973	1974	1975
Manufacturing industry	3540	3520	3710	3520	3490
	(4.3)	(3.9)	(4.2)	(4.5)	(3.7)
Construction	3570	3650	3540	3330	3530
	(19.6)	(18.7)	(21.6)	(16.0)	(18.1)
Railways and railway employment	2830	2790	3010	2770	2920
	(24.1)	(19.7)	(18.3)	(14.8)	(18.7)
Coal mining	26090	20470	24630	19310	20940
	(24.2)	(22.1)	(29.6)	(18.7)	(24.7)
Quarries	6010	5930	4510	3730	3770
	(47.4)	(40.7)	(29.0)	(31.2)	(30.1)
Agriculture			1970	1890	1800
			(14.7)	(10.9)	(11.7)

Note: [a]Fatality incidence is shown in brackets.
Source: *Health and Safety Statistics 1975* (HSE, HMSO)

If, in addition to the changing balance of the workforce, we also consider the contraction that has taken place in the total numbers employed in all the sectors shown in Table 7.2, it is probable that the degree of risk in these sectors, as measured by incidence rates, is as high currently as at any time in the post-war period.

Part of the reason for this is to be found in the mounting numbers of workplace hazards that have been produced as an unfortunate consequence of technical progress. Toxic substances are a prime example and emphasise the importance of occupational health service provision both to cope with and evaluate the effects of such substances on the workforce. The Deputy Chief Inspector of Factories recently estimated that approximately 4 million new chemicals have been identified in the last ten years and that currently between 20 and 30 thousand chemicals are manufactured worldwide in quantities greater than one ton per annum. The total number of dangerous substances in use in industry and their long-term effects on exposed workers are simply not known.

Our knowledge of long-term health risks extends to only a fraction of those substances in common use in industry. Moreover, in the absence of extensive and effective epidemiological monitoring of workers exposed to various toxic substances — a task which could incidentally be carried out by a comprehensive occupational health service — the accuracy of statistics relating to deaths resulting from industrial diseases and workplace exposure must be strongly open to question.

At the end of 1976 the Employment Medical Advisory Service employed some 200 doctors and nurses (Health and Safety Commission 1977). These apart, it has been estimated that 600 full-time doctors work in occupational health services backed up by around 4000 part-timers, mostly local GPs with little or no occupational health training. It is further estimated that for half of the working population — around 11 million people — no work-based medical cover exists at all. In the last section we turn to examine how this wholly inadequate provision could be radically improved.

The NHS and Occupational Health Service Provision

It is the inescapable conclusion of this chapter that only as an integrated part of the NHS can we hope to provide a medical service to those at work comparable to that called for by the TUC in 1944. Having said this, it is equally clear that neither simple nor short-term means are available to bring about this end.

As a logical first step however, all existing full-time personnel working in occupational health services could be 'taken over' by the state. That is they should become employed by, paid by, trained by and accountable to the NHS. This would go a long way towards removing the firmly held suspicion that as long as factory doctors are paid by the company they are essentially company men influenced by corporate goals and values. It can be argued that it is in the factory doctors' interest for this particular relationship to be severed.

The extent to which a company doctor's medical judgement may be compromised by an equal awareness of his employer's commercial priorities was well illustrated in the case of Stokes v GKN (Bolts and Nuts) Ltd. In this case a worker died of scrotal cancer contracted from oil-soaked overalls. The factory doctor knew of the risk but decided not to warn the workforce lest it should worry them unnecessarily. The judge in the case decided that the doctor's actions to 'soothe' rather than 'alert' were wrong and that he had a duty to warn employees of the risk. Currently factory doctors taking similar courses of action may find themselves liable to prosecution under Section 7 of the Health and

Safety at Work Act, 1974 for failing

> to take reasonable care for the health and safety of himself and of
> other persons who may be affected by his acts or omissions at
> work . . .

Moreover, it would seem axiomatic that medical judgements and
decisions within industry should be formed completely independently
of other management priorities.

The financing of an occupational health service as an arm of the
NHS (particularly in the current fiscal climate) might be thought to be
an intractable problem. However, there would seem to be no real reason
why the necessary funds could not be raised from industry (which
will after all directly benefit from the service) via a compulsory levy
along the lines of that which currently maintains and operates the
various Industrial Training Boards.

The real problems may not be so fundamentally economic but
rather related to our ability to train and service an expanded body of
permanent and peripatetic occupational health personnel. The EMAS
survey showed a very low level of specialised training amongst occupational health service personnel. Of the doctors employed full-time, 42
per cent had either the Diploma in Industrial Health (DIH) or the MSC
in occupational medicine but, over all, including part-time doctors, less
than 20 per cent possess any special qualifications. The position was
found to be broadly similar for factory nurses: about 20 per cent were
found to possess the Occupational Health Nursing Certificate (OHNC).

Occupational medicine is very poorly represented in basic medical
education, quite apart from specialist postgraduate training. The recent
survey of undergraduate medical training (General Medical Council
1977) suggests that at most medical schools all aspects of 'community
medicine' are granted a fairly minor place, and within that occupational
and industrial medicine seem to receive little attention at all but five
medical schools. The Royal Commission on Medical Education (1968)
did little to encourage expanded training in this area. The Report
remarked that there would be little need for industrial health services in
the future. Their reasoning was a classic self-fulfilling prophecy (para.
52, p. 39):

> The main reason for this does not, we think, lie in the pattern of
> employment or the nature of the relationship between employer and
> employee in this country, but rather in the fact that this country has

given first priority to the establishment of a comprehensive system of medical services fully available to all sections of the community. The existence of such a system must limit the scope of the services demanded of British industrial medicine, and we do not expect any major changes in this respect in the foreseeable future.

A priority must be to increase the numbers of specially trained personnel flowing into industry which in turn requires a higher priority being afforded to this aspect of medical training in hospitals and university departments. Whilst desirable, it must be recognised that such an achievement will inevitably take time. However, some short-run strategies to boost trained personnel and increase resource utilisation could and should be considered. The Health and Safety Commission in their consultative document on occupational health services make three suggestions that merit urgent consideration: (a) the extension to smaller neighbours of the occupational health services of larger firms; (b) the joint provision of specialised occupational health services for firms within the same industry; (c) the boosting of local occupational health services run by trained occupational health nurses.

The first two ideas could be developed and co-ordinated in association with local NHS hospital facilities, perhaps utilising peripatetic staff to ensure contact between hospital-based and factory-based medical staff. It is suggested that this type of relationship would help to foster a greater awareness and understanding of industrial conditions and health hazards amongst hospital-based staff.

The third development obviously requires careful examination since our basic goal must be the provision of the best possible service to industry. However, it may be that properly trained occupational health nurses, given the appropriate backing from neighbouring company services and local NHS facilities, could provide an efficient service to many firms.

A further argument for state control over occupational health services can be found in the type of activity most frequently carried out by existing voluntary services. The EMAS survey showed that:

Treatment is the activity most frequently carried out, with emergency treatment being the most common. Pre-employment medical examinations are also carried out by most services. Activities concerned with the prevention of disease and/or injury are less common and this is particularly noticeable in the case of those preventative activities which require special expertise or facilities such as epidemiology, medical examinations to detect unrecognised hazards or environmental surveillance to detect hazards emanating from the site.

Yet as this chapter has sought to demonstrate, it is vital that we should be able to move occupational health services beyond just treatment to a more positive, preventive role. Treatment alone, though necessary, is not a sufficient condition for the control of technological and post-industrial hazards of work. There is no doubt that the newer industrial hazards require detailed, dispassionate monitoring and assessment, which calls for resources, expertise and training well beyond that which is provided by the vast majority of voluntary services. Further-more, it is submitted that only a state-controlled service could provide the necessary freedom from commercial priorities to enable the effec-tive monitoring of hazards to be carried out.

Currently, accidents and injuries sustained at work, at a conservative estimate, reach the annual equivalent cost of one per cent of GNP. Days lost from accidents at work alone averaged 16.8 million per annum between 1970 and 1975 — many times more than the equivalent number of days lost through industrial disputes (see Gregory and McCarty 1975). The degree of individual pain and suffering cannot be quantified. Against this the relevance of the NHS seems to be clear, as do the choices facing us as a society. On the one hand, we can maintain the existing confusion of state and voluntary services, leaving as many as half of the workforce scandalously underprovided for. On the other hand we could, as a society, recognise the validity of the call voiced by the TUC over 30 years ago and provide a genuine occupational health service as part of the NHS and in so doing make a real contribution to the quality of life both in and outside work.

8 HIDDEN LABOUR AND THE NATIONAL HEALTH SERVICE

Jane Taylor

At this time of economic crisis and severe constraints on public expenditure we are witnessing the redrawing of the boundaries between curative and caring services, institutional and domiciliary services, paid and unpaid labour. The setting up of the Royal Commission on the NHS and the recent statements contained in *The Way Forward* (DHSS 1977c) are part of a process of redefining what kinds of need can and should be met by the health service, and what kinds of need should be met through social services, volunteer help, and care provided by the families and friends of those in need. We are witnessing not simply a shift of resources away from the acute medical sector to other services but a change in the very forms of labour and collectivised care. It appears that one form of labour — paid, trained, often expensive, based in institutions — is being replaced by other forms of labour — low paid, or unpaid, untrained and seemingly cheap. The justifications for this strategy come in two major guises: that it is both inefficient and undesirable to provide institutional care through the NHS for large numbers of the mentally ill, mentally handicapped, and chronically sick; and that the 'home' and 'family' if given proper support constitute a better caring environment. In this contribution the central question is whether the strategy, contained in *The Way Forward*, of extending the role of domiciliary and unpaid care through informal networks is either feasible or desirable. This question is vitally important for women. It is their unpaid labour in the home, as carers, nurses, cooks, which represents a vast quantity of care on which the selective provision of welfare services is predicated.

How far are policies aimed at 'helping families to care' based on realistic expectations of the quality and quantity of care that can be provided from informal, and unpaid sources? It is possible that current pressures to increase NHS efficiency, to intensify the use of facilities and to shift care into the community, may result in a sharp deterioration in the standards of care provided both inside and outside the NHS. It is important then to consider how far the 'community' can care and how far unpaid, privatised, and invisible care does meet the needs of dependent individuals. Clearly questions about the extent and signifi-

cance of this hidden care and the degree to which it could be substituted for institutional welfare services and waged personnel are both
political and emotive. It is important to debate the possible impact of
DHSS policy on those fulfilling caring roles and on the different categories of people in need of treatment, nursing and support.

The 'Priorities' Document (DHSS 1976c) and *The Way Forward*
present themselves as a response to changing morbidity and mortality
patterns, to the growth in the numbers of elderly people and the special
problems they present. But they contain numerous assumptions about
the nature of care in the home and in the community which suggest
that the DHSS has attached insufficient weight to changes in the position of women and the possible implications of their present employment patterns for traditional caring roles. We need to look at these
assumptions, the position of women and the increase in chronic need
(due to ageing and degenerative diseases) in order to assess just what
The Way Forward means for the balance between collectively provided
services, and those provided invisibly and privately. Only a beginning
can be made here.

Caring in the Home and Community

The family is an important source of care and support in our society
and for many in need it constitutes a 'first line of defence'. While the
welfare state provides a wide range of services to meet specific needs, a
high value has been placed on non-collective care and on maintaining
mutual kinship obligations in the event of old age, illness and dependence. The creation of the NHS removed one set of specific needs from
the sphere of the family, the unprofessional carer and the volunteer,
and redefined them as the responsibility of collectively provided professional services. But the 'Cinderella' sectors of care, such as the
mentally ill, the mentally handicapped and the elderly, have remained
heavily dependent on the unpaid and non-professional care given by
families and neighbours.

This privatised, hidden labour has received little social or monetary
recognition. Social security and taxation provisions have taken little
note of the specific needs of the non-able bodied and many rely on
basic Supplementary Benefit. The Constant Attendance Allowance
(1971) and the new Invalid Care Allowance do represent an important
step towards acknowledging that care for the mentally handicapped or
invalids is a form of work in which carers incur costs and that these
costs should be reimbursed through a collectively provided cash benefit.

In recent years the Women's Liberation Movement has drawn atten-

tion to the privatised domestic labour of women. Several feminist
writers have begun to question why this labour receives so little direct
reward and why women in their families have been expected by governments and policy makers to take on caring roles, often at great social
and psychological costs to themselves. What began as an attempt by
these writers to make visible the invisible, to expose and define the
isolation of the housewife, has now developed into analyses of the
separation of the private sphere of the home and the social sphere of
production (e.g. Gardiner 1976). The existence of collectively provided
welfare services has been seen as standing between the two spheres: the
services transform some previously unpaid caring tasks into wage
labour and meet selected needs. But the distinction between wage
labour and unpaid domestic labour is maintained − the housewife cum
nurse, cook, childminder, is not rewarded in the same way as someone
performing these same tasks in a 'real' job − and individuals and
families are expected to meet many of their needs themselves. Collective provision is thus premised on concepts of family responsibility and
domestic labour.

Zaretsky (1976), Gardiner and others have tried to illustrate the
process whereby work in the home came to be seen as not 'real' work,
because it lay outside commodity exchange. They suggest that work
performed in the family has been defined as emotional, caring activities
which cannot be reduced to a monetary dimension. Moroney (1976),
for example, argues that professional, collectively provided care has
only been made available where the individual in need and his/her relatives are quite unable to meet the need according to the judgement of a
professional or welfare agent, e.g. a doctor, or health visitor. He suggests
that care by friends and family has often been seen as morally superior
to care provided through the cash nexus. From a feminist point of view,
however, this privatised domestic labour has meant economic dependence, social isolation and low social status for many women. A number
of feminist writers have provided strident critiques of this dependence
and the ideological content of concepts such as 'home' and 'family'.
Oakley (1974b), Davidoff *et al.* (1976), Brunsdon (1978) and others
argue that the 'home' and the sphere of the family emerged as the
sphere of emotional and supportive relationships in the context of industrialisation. The home became a sphere set apart from the dehumanisation and powerlessness experienced in wage labour. The home came
to offer opportunities for private control over the pace of work and
over relationships. But at the same time it became defined as the sphere
in which woman's natural 'femininity' and her ability to nurse, minister

and care could flourish. Femininity thus becomes synonymous with tenderness, love and care: true womanhood becomes defined as the fulfilment of the needs and desires of others and 'home' emerges as the sphere of personal freedom and basic human values:

> Femininity is defined by the intimate relations of the family . . . whereas men reproduce themselves through their industry, women reproduce themselves almost entirely through these interpersonal relations. Thus women experience themselves as a response to other people's needs – most importantly their emotional needs . . . because a woman's activity is invested in people rather than objects. (Foreman 1977:102)

How far can one argue, though, that social policies have reflected this kind of conceptualisation of the personal sphere and women's roles within it? Is it valid to suggest, as Jordan (1976) does, that welfare policies have generally been intended to 'enhance the sense of family responsibility' and the caring roles of women? One way to begin to consider this question is to look briefly at the assumptions and objectives which have underpinned health service policy. It is only possible here to focus briefly on selected aspects of policy development. The policies for 'community care' which have been described as part-hopes and part-descriptions are used as an example.

Policies for community care stem from the 1959 Mental Health Act and the Royal Commission on mental illness and mental handicap which preceded the Act. The main concern behind the Act was to close down the old, often ex Poor Law institutions for the mentally ill and to reduce the total numbers of long-stay patients. It was argued that such institutions had a debilitating effect on some patients and that many inmates did not require expensive medical care in an institutional setting. The objective of reducing capital expenditure and freeing blocked beds was thus attractive economically and supported by research on institutionalisation. It was hoped that the drug revolution in tranquillisers would open up the possibility of more short-term admissions and a shift in emphasis towards care provided in the community, through hostels, home helps, day care centres and relatives. It is significant that the intention was that care should no longer focus solely on the individual but on the individual living in a network of social relations. Implicit in the 1959 Act was the assumption that families and friends with 'support' from community-based services could provide highly labour-intensive care for large numbers of mentally ill and mentally handicapped people. Both the Act and the subsequent 1962 Hospital Plan emphasised that the role of NHS hospitals had to be the treatment of medical needs and the provision of cures where possible: it was both wasteful and inappropriate for the NHS to provide long-term care for certain categories of mental illness.

Since 1959 definitions of 'community care' have been extended to include everything from outpatient care to community hospital services to informal lay care. But through the Act, the Seebohm Report (1968) and the two White Papers on mental illness and mental handicap (DHSS 1971 and 1975) one can trace a strong commitment to non-institutional care and to the mobilisation and encouragement of unpaid care by relatives and volunteers. It is suggested that it is inherently undesirable to segregate such patients from their families and communities and that these families can and should provide care in ordinary private homes. The crucial question here must concern the justifiability of arguing that the home environment has the potential to provide good quality care at low cost, even with minimal support from statutory services.

Policies for community care are characterised by a desire to contain costs and demand in the welfare state and by implicit assumptions about the home as a caring environment. We lack sufficient research and information to judge accurately just how families, individuals and carers do cope with the needs which are otherwise met by 24 hour institutional care. But one can suggest that some approaches to community care display romantic images of families and community as caring agents. Lapping (1970) comments that 'community care' hints at 'Arcadian villages' caring for their 'oddballs' and argues

> When we talk of community care we are employing a linguistic sleight of hand. What it often means is care by an individual family for a sick member for whom at one time the whole community — through a hospital — might have taken responsibility.

She suggests that such care can mean little more than the 'sum of individual burdens' — burdens which have to be borne privately precisely because the reduction in hospital beds, the rise in short-term hospital admissions (especially amongst the mentally ill) and the highly selective provision of welfare services in the community leaves no alternative. Presumably as Moroney (1976) has argued, many families 'cope' but we do not know how adequately they cope and at what cost. Moroney cites Maddox (1975):

A family does not always provide a benign environment for its members. Parents do not always want the children they bear; they are not always capable of providing the resources necessary for their development as healthy competent individuals . . . Adult children do not always, and cannot always assume responsibility for their ageing parents. Families are thus sometimes the source of problems for their members; and the resources which families can and will make available to members are limited.

The Seebohm Report, the 1971 and 1975 White Papers and the Priorities' document do recognise that informal or family care for the elderly, chronic sick or mentally ill has limits depending on the level and type of need. At the same time, it is assumed that some extension of non-institutional, supportive services will mean that families and individuals will find 'allies' enabling them to realise their potential for care. This raises an interesting dilemma in the relationship between collective and privatised care. The personal, private sphere of the home is both morally superior and, due to the hidden costs of domestic labour, cheap in comparison with professionalised institutional provision. Yet it cannot be assumed that care will automatically be provided within this sphere in a way which is defined as appropriate by policy makers and welfare agents. While caring is both natural and legitimate within the sphere of home and community, it has simultaneously to be nurtured, encouraged and supported. Wilson (1977) argues that this relationship between paid welfare agents and unpaid carers is a relationship of exploitation and coercion which has to be understood in terms of how the welfare state 'serves the needs of Capital'. In her view the combined effect of the structure and level of provision of health and social services enforces and imposes caring relationships between families and neighbours – at a huge hidden cost to all involved.

To clarify some of these issues we need to look at the information we do have on care in the community – its scope, quality, complexity and costs, whether social, psychological or financial. The future potential of such care then needs to be set in the wider social context of changes in demography, need and community structure. One might then be in a position to assess whether the concepts of manipulation, exploitation and romanticism (used by critics of community care such as Wilson and Jordan) are in fact useful in an analysis of unpaid and voluntary care.

Who Can Care?

Much of the research on how volunteers, neighbours and families cope with caring for the sick, handicapped and disturbed in the home has focused on particular client groups. Very little work has been done from a feminist perspective. Moroney brings together data from a wide range of sources, but as he points out, there are enormous gaps in our knowledge of informal and unpaid care. Others have shown some of the social and psychological costs to carers and dependents, where care is provided with little collective provision; their work highlights the sheer volume of labour borne privately. Bayley (1973) for example, describes the 'social euthanasia' and hardship which can occur where families (usually the mother of the mentally handicapped people that he studied) provide long-term, intensive care. He points out that the lack of supportive services may mean that the carer may be placed under the same restrictions as in looking after a child under five − but in the case of the mentally handicapped care may be provided for a lifetime. Bayley emphasises the desirability of strengthening families' ability and willingness to care, but he comments

> Community care for the chronically handicapped has got by largely by exploiting the families of handicapped people. But for the care given by families and friends, many of these people would be in hospital. If they were, care would be provided twenty-four hours a day. The care of those at home needs to be considered in the same terms.

Abrams (1977) echoes a similar concern to this when he comments:

> If we could find a language for translating psychological costs into cash terms it is almost certain that community care would prove a great deal more expensive than institutional care.

They both suggest that greater social recognition should be given to such privatised care. As several commentators have pointed out though, greater social and financial acknowledgement of this care would be very expensive for the welfare state, since this labour is at present carried out by the 'largest unpaid sector of society'. In short, the work of Meacher, Bayley and others shows that patients and clients who do receive professional, collectively provided care represent only a fraction of those who potentially need support and help. Their work shows the problems that arise where families or individuals are not able to provide good quality care — and where care in the 'home environment' does not necessarily compensate for the lack of professional help and the lack of resources to meet the dependent person's needs.

The amount of unmet and unrecognised need is always a thorny question in discussions on social policy: we can however look at the level of demand on existing services and at changing morbidity, mortality and demographic data. This allows us to estimate approximately what level of service has to be provided in order to provide the same *real* level of care relative to changing need. What would be relevant, for example, would be changes in the ratio of home helps to the elderly population rather than absolute changes in the numbers of either group. If we look at the balance of care provided by the institutional and community health services and at the rates of growth in these services, it does appear that there has been a shift away from institutional care for several categories of need without a commensurate increase in forms of community care that would maintain constant let alone improved *real* levels of care.

> While the explicit policy since 1959 may have emphasized community services, experience since then suggests that the policy is less than meaningful . . . Demand for the domiciliary services has increased faster than resources and recipients are being provided less services than in the past, whether this is the number of hours per week of home help and home nursing or the number of meals per week. Accompanying this is a trend among providers of service to establish priorities among potential users. Elderly people who live alone or just with their spouses are more likely to receive services while those who live with their children or within an extended kin network are more likely to be denied help. (Moroney 1976:58)

When placed alongside first the low targets proposed in *The Way Forward* for the expansion of domiciliary services, to meet the needs of the growing numbers of elderly and chronic sick, and second the move towards short-term institutional provision for both the physically and mentally ill, these trends lend weight to the argument that unpaid and unskilled care is of fundamental and growing importance in the welfare state.

The extent to which such care can be provided and to what standard has to be a historically specific question. The 'family' or 'community' are social phenomena which continually change and evolve: just as wage labour is dynamic and historically specific, so labour in the home changes with the nature of its tasks and the available resources. The experience and the labour of the modern housewife caring for an ageing parent or a mentally handicapped child is not the same as her predecessors in past decades. In the past two decades we have seen dramatic changes in the structure of families and households which have important implications for social policy. The number of married women working has risen, family size has declined and the number of households containing only one or two people has risen. (Between 1951 and 1971 the proportion in this category rose from 38 per cent to 49 per cent of all households.) This is due to the compression of fertility, the fact that young people leave home at an earlier age and that more elderly people live apart from their kin. Geographical mobility has undermined some of the functions previously performed through extended family networks. These trends have alarming implications as we move rapidly towards a 'mass elderly society' and a situation where the ratio between working life and post working life is rising steadily. At the same time the rise in the numbers of married women working and a decline in what Moroney has termed the 'caretaker pool' of women aged 45-60 who have traditionally provided a tremendous amount of care for the ageing, sick and non-able bodied raises doubts over how far adequate care for those in need can be provided outside the welfare services, or with low level support from the latter. With more women in the labour force, with fewer spinsters and rising numbers of elderly, who is going to care?

It is true that much of the rise in women's employment has been in part-time work and that women workers have continued to occupy a vulnerably and often low-paid position in the labour market. Women workers in the NHS reflect this: it is no accident that the NHS as a highly labour-intensive service has relied heavily on low-paid, female and immigrant labour, and on part-time labour. These trends in employment and family structure raise two important types of questions concerning the provision of care both within the NHS and outside it. First, how far can women — who in the past have borne the brunt of care for dependents — continue to fulfil dual roles as part-time workers and domestic labourers? Does the expansion of part-time work in fact imply that women and families will continue to provide a lot of care for the elderly, and other groups, with little collective support? Secondly, we have seen hospital workers in recent months struggling to protect their jobs and the quality of care provided, in the face of resource constraints and faster 'throughput' of patients. But who will struggle to protect the quality of care given in the private and personal sphere, in the 'community' at large? What future role can we expect and should we construct for voluntary and non-collective provision of care?

Questions such as these cannot be answered pragmatically and empirically in terms of, for example, the targets to be set for the ratio of day centre places to numbers of elderly and infirm people. The issues are more fundamental than that. They centre on three axes: what should be the future allocation of rewards between different kinds of labour? who should have the power to decide what resources and collectively provided services are available to the non-able bodied, on what terms? what should be the balance between collective and privatised provision of care? It is perhaps helpful to make explicit some of the ideological and political issues at stake here, by looking briefly at recent radical critiques of NHS and welfare policies.

Theories of the Welfare State

Several recent socialist feminist analyses of the welfare state have argued that it is highly improbable that there will be any major extension in collective provision for the non-able bodied. In thier view welfare services represent a very limited collectivisation of care within a hierarchical and authoritarian framework: recipients of care and their families have little control over the services. Some analyses suggest that a fundamental characteristic of capitalism is the perpetuation of women's roles as domestic labourers, so that the burden of care and reproduction (washing, cleaning, childminding etc.) is borne privately and women may be exploited as a flexible 'reserve army' of wage labour. This approach tends to explain social policies — for example the 'efficiency' movement in the NHS — in terms of the need of capital to limit public expenditure, containing demands on the welfare state, through ideologies about individualism and 'family responsibilities'. Critics who adopt this perspective argue that privatised reproduction is a central feature of women's oppression under capitalism. For both economic and ideological reasons it is inconceivable that the welfare state will collectivise more than a fraction of this labour. The very existence of wage labour available to capital on favourable terms is predicated on the existence of a mass of domestic labour, which is not directly rewarded and which is carried out in numerous privatised units.

Wilson's approach to social policies places a greater emphasis on ideology and the social control function of welfare provision. She maintains that the enforcement of family responsibilities has been fundamental to the 'purposes of welfarism'. In her view welfare agencies have manipulated and monitored the performance of caring roles in the home and community. The deviant family or individual who fails to meet their 'proper' responsibilities unaided is liable to face a descending army of social workers — or the alternative of low-standard institutional care for the aged, mentally ill and mentally handicapped. She argues that when welfare agents 'help' women and individuals to cope with illness or stress they are literally forcing unpaid domestic labourers to do a job for the capitalist state. Jordan's analysis is similar in some respects: like Wilson he argues that Poor Law principles still operate to ensure that the able bodied do take responsibility for their non-able bodied dependents. Moroney (1976) provides one instance of this process when he describes the extent to which families are expected to care for elderly kin: where a kin network is believed to exist, help may be withheld.

The above analyses are provocative and polemical but they do attempt a theoretical analysis of the existing divisions between collective and privatised care. They contradict the view that the struggle to improve welfare services is fundamentally a struggle for 'more of the same' — more hospitals, more doctors, more caring agents. And by discussing the 'oppressive' features of privatised reproduction they raise the questions about the forms of collective provision which might be developed. It is important to emphasise though, that these kinds of approach to social policy have tended to oversimplify many of the issues. The 'family' and the 'state' are often posed as two entities locked into a relationship of exploitation. In the context of health services this dichotomy obscures the wide range of care provided through voluntary organisations and other informal networks — and the positive value that many people attach to these sources of care. The issue is not really care by the family *or* the state, since 'individual burdens' can be shared through a variety of means, potentially under the control of those using networks of care. Second, many feminist discussions of welfare provision have centred on the care of children, and on the need to expand institutional facilities and to raise cash benefits like Child Benefits, in recognition of the labour involved in childrearing. There has been a tendency to focus on relationships between parents and children and to neglect many of the relationships between adults, which involve long-term dependence and care. More attention needs to be paid to what fully socialised health care would mean in practice: would it mean simply greater institutional provision and the creation of new benefits parallel to Child Benefits for those caring for the sick outside the NHS? One could argue that neither of these approaches would necessarily be in the interests of dependents or carers. Third, at their worst the analyses briefly outlined above represent a new combination of conspiracy theory and functionalism: a personified monolithic capitalist state manipulates, exploits and controls: it launches 'ideological offensives' against women in order to press them back into the home and into caring roles, when they are no longer needed in the labour force. At times these analyses suggest a very mechanistic approach to policy making and the provision of services: this enables one to gloss over the positive values attached to family life and the unpaid provision of care, where these can mean privacy, independence and personal satisfaction.

Which Way Forward?

Do any of the above approaches help provide a basis on which to criticise the DHSS's *The Way Forward* and on which to formulate alternative strategies? Both the Priorities Document and *The Way Forward* assume that only a very limited increase in resources will be available to expand collective services. Thus, within a limited budget, resources must be redeployed away from the acute medical sector in order to expand domiciliary services in response to the growing numbers of elderly and chronic sick. But given the targets set for the expansion of home helps, day centre places and the time it is anticipated it will take to achieve them it is open to question whether even the current real levels of provision will be protected. The DHSS's insistence that the targets represent only 'purely illustrative projections' which Local Authorities may deviate from or ignore does not give one grounds for confidence. For example, officers of the Personal Social Services Council commented on *The Way Forward* with dismay:

> We are prompted to ask how authorities are to achieve the objective of maintaining standards of care in a situation where the number of very elderly people is increasing rapidly, the real level of residential provision and of hospital in-patient services is going down, the development of community hospitals is likely to be slower than previously envisaged, there is no corresponding increase in the rates of growth proposed for the community health services, and the proposed increase in projected expenditure on the fieldwork and domiciliary services seems not to be happening.

The policy of putting 'people before buildings' may turn out in practice to mean reductions in 'priority' services such as meals on wheels or home nurses, and increasing pressure on hospital beds and staff — where 'efficiency' is being equated with increasing cases per bed — reducing average lengths of stay in hospital and discharging patients as quickly as possible to the care provided in their own homes, often by hard-pressed and untrained relatives. Given the low targets set for expansion of domiciliary services one can anticipate that, for some non-able bodied, care provided by trained, skilled personnel is gradually going to be replaced by care provided by less-trained, lower-paid, or unpaid individuals. And while it is possible that the DHSS's hopes for volunteer labour can be realised it is worth pointing out that care by unspecialised, lay members of the community has been described as 'typically volatile, spasmodic, and unreliable; very much not a social fact' (Abrams 1977).

The DHSS's *Way Forward* is based on a consistent set of assumptions concerning the relationship between collective and privatised care. It is assumed that resources available for collective care are very limited. Therefore it is necessary to limit the expansion in the number of wage labourers in caring roles at present carried out by unpaid labourers (hence low targets for the number of home helps and so forth): in addition, if, as feared, collective provision does not keep in step with the rising numbers of elderly, then privatised care will have to expand. This is partly what Wilson (1977) means when she refers to the crisis in capitalism and constraints on public expenditure as intensifying the 'exploitation' of women. Needs are defined as potentially infinite and as expanding in response to a greater supply of welfare services. Hence the DHSS insists that the welfare state can only meet a limited range of needs, and families and volunteers can and should provide an amount of care which far outstrips what is provided collectively.

The assumptions which underpin the DHSS's *Way Forward* reflect not only the very real and immediate problems it faces in budgeting for welfare services but also wider views in our society of the way in which different forms of labour should be rewarded and resources distributed.

The present distribution of wealth and income is based on a set of values which give little recognition to caring roles or to private labour in the home. If the distinction between what is now privatised domestic labour and wage labour broke down it would entail a huge redistribution of income between different kinds of work and a transformation in social values. Socialist feminists have argued that this could only occur in a transition to socialism, where the present separation between the social and the private sphere broke down.

However, such analyses do not provide one with more pragmatic and short-term means of improving care. Does this mean that, with minor modifications, one has to accept the DHSS strategy as the only one which is both feasible and economic, in the current situation? Or should we be looking beyond the present forms of welfare provision to innovations such as new cash benefits to reward lay care (e.g. Constant Attendance Allowance for those caring for mentally handicapped) or to methods of promoting voluntary organisation and reciprocal self-help amongst groups in need. The introduction of new benefits such as the Constant Attendance Allowance and the Invalid Care Allowance do represent a recognition of previously unpaid labour. But the payment of such benefits provides no guarantee of the quality of care provided and it can be argued that such benefits will in principle perpetuate the isolated, privatised nature of care by relatives and lay people. Abrams has argued that the introduction of such cash benefits, or the development of Good Neighbour schemes where cash incentives are used, may both commercialise caring relationships and erode informal, if erratic, mutual aid between kin, neighbours and friends. If this occurred the need for welfare services and cash incentives would increase – and this would involve heavier expenditure. One can turn this argument round and suggest firstly, that it is mistaken to define costs to the welfare state – in cash terms – as the most important consideration since this undervalues the hidden costs to individuals when collective provision is *not* made. Secondly, the possible erosion of informal care that Abrams fears must be set in context: a mass of informal care and domestic labour lies outside the cash nexus and receives little social recognition. But this is not a reason to limit the provision of financial and other material rewards for this labour, so much as to make it visible as an important form of work and to challenge the present allocation of rewards and status between those working in the 'private sphere' and those involved in social production.

Finally, Moroney, Townsend and other commentators have emphasised the potential role that volunteers could play in meeting need. In recent years, the DHSS has certainly increased its support for voluntary organisations. With the disappearance of the enclosed, interdependent communities which used to provide often extensive and effective care for many and with the changes in family structure mentioned above, it seems questionable how far volunteers can be a source of care which is both reliable and 'inexpensive'.

'Hidden labour' will it seems continue to underpin the whole edifice of welfare state provision in *The Way Forward*. This is due to three major limitations in the DHSS approach. First, a failure to question fundamentally the distribution of rewards for different kinds of labour.

Second, a failure to redefine radically the value to be attached to the care of the non able-bodied and dependent. Third, an evasion of the issue of how control over services and resources could shift from professionals and state employees to the clients, their friends, neighbours and kin making use of collectively provided resources. To achieve the fuller socialisation of care for dependent people, change in all three of these areas would be essential, in order to transform hundreds of individual burdens into collective responsibilities.

9 PRACTISING HEALTH CARE: THE NURSE PRACTITIONER

Rita Austin

If prevention and health is *everybody's* business does this necessitate any re-alignment of position between doctors, patients, nurses, therapists and other paramedical workers? (DHSS 1976a, 1977d). If prevention and health is *everybody's* business is it then not *somebody's* particular business? And if it is somebody's particular business, who should that somebody be? Is it to be a doctor who may be trained to deal with management of illness, or a health visitor whose training contains far greater emphasis on prevention and on promotion of positive health? More important, is the rationale and structure of the organisation of health services geared to cure and care of the sick, the same as one geared more toward promotion of health? This essay is devoted to exploration of the idea and ethos of a nurse practitioner, arguing that this is better suited to the practice of health care than the current medically oriented work arrangements and practices.

Health and Illness

Models of contemporary health care practice are grounded in notions of medical cure. Consequently this has meant a predominant emphasis on the medical model as the preferred form of treatment and the medical practitioner as the epitome of professional service. Furthermore the impact on provision and practice is such that neither the National, Health or Service promised by that title is fulfilled. Not for nothing has the National Health Service come to be known as the National Sickness Service. It is worth noting that such a title is not merely a description. While the description is accurate, there are punning undertones. That is to say, the accurately described National Sickness Service is itself far from 'well'. This may be because of an excessive bureaucratisation so that the means of achieving ends become so important that they obscure those ends. Or it may be that inter-professional tensions invalidate the contribution of each individual profession. Whichever it is need not detain us unduly here. Suffice it to say that the twin impact of bureaucracy and profession on a health service oriented toward cure have done little to procure health care and much to exacerbate the sickness of a service for the sick.

145

A remarkable feature of current thinking about the National Health Service is the consistent attack made upon it. The attack is manifest in criticism of the efficacy of contemporary health care provision. The inherent nature of recurring capital and labour costs in the service is at last understood as never before. Whether critics favour 'free' provision of health care or not, all recognise that the medical maw of treatment is both self-perpetuating and by definition insatiable. There has also been a much wider appreciation of the radical changes that have come to pass in the health care needs of contemporary post-industrial societies. Changes, for example, in the age structure of the population, in the incidence and nature of disease, in the stress complaints brought about by the pace of modern urban life. Changes which, less tangibly, but with equal force, have affected the consciousness of a people so that they are encouraged to look to the specialists to define (and then to treat) health care needs. Obesity, anxiety and some forms of depression are cases in point. It is also recognised that this state of affairs is exacerbated by family and wider social structures which inhibit opportunity even were there the will to take charge of health. Small nuclear families separated from kin and living in houses ill adapted to caring for the dis-ease which not unnaturally accompanies stages in the life cycle, are themselves ill at ease in providing for the health care needs of family members who may be old, mentally or physically disabled or just periodically incapable of carrying out their usual social roles.

Providers and consumers alike of the NHS are becoming increasingly aware of the dysfunctions of bureaucracy and profession in the Service and more importantly coming round to the view that, bureaucracy and profession apart, even the neutral impact of medical intervention (if such were possible) on the health of a society is not as efficacious as it might be. That is, that the health of a nation is not completely served by what medicine can do and that this stage of wellness is probably more dependent on the provision of non-medical supports like good housing, non-polluted environments, adequate nutritional levels, physical exercise, stress-alleviating interpersonal relationships, minimum income levels, job satisfaction and so on. Wilson's comment is apposite:

> There is no way to health through the cure of illness. Indeed we can no longer maintain the old *clinical* distinction between 'wellness' and 'illness' upon which the Health Service is based. Rather than trying to reach health by understanding illness, we must first try to understand health, in the light of which we may be able to say something

about being well or ill. (Wilson 1975)

The Value of Health

This shift of mood and thought among health care commentators (and increasingly practitioners) is towards a view of health as being related to what people believe is the fullest life for them, i.e. as situational. The efficacy of modern surgery and medical care has banished the basis for the Victorians' preoccupation with death. Now that survival is more assured, attention can be concentrated on the quality of life. If anything, an appreciable segment of the contemporary view of health maintains that the intensity with which we hold to the value of medical intervention of itself underdevelops a people's capacity to take charge of their own health.

Our situational view of health is far removed from the Victorian in relation to the medical cure of acute disease, but, paradoxically, the Victorian endeavour in relation to the control of environmental hazards is being renewed in the contemporary health value placed on prevention. Clearly the points of departure are dissimilar as one would expect in an industrialising society and a post-industrial one, but the thrust and general orientation of today's health value mirrors the Victorian ideal. This is something to which I shall return having made the point here that because health is an expression of what people value (see Murcott in this volume), and because in a world of limited resources choice must be made between competing valued goods and services, the endeavour to build a healthy society is an art involving ethical and political considerations. Health, then, is better seen as a public creation and not wholly a private specialism, however scientific. Sol Tax makes an additional point which is worth mentioning here to counteract the widely held belief that our present health service orientations and work arrangements are immutable. He remarks that in as much as disease is influenced by socio-cultural systems, so are means of maintaining the health of individuals. His final comment deserves note:

> Although much in illness is universal and biological, the health system in any culture is as artificial and changeable as anything else in human society. (Tax 1975)

As I shall attempt to demonstrate, this situational construction of health cannot be simply accomplished. No one profession's definition of health will suffice, nor will the domination of health care practice by one profession. Neither will the straightforward cumulation of personal health practices of the do-it-yourself variety and series of publicly dispensed exhortations serve any more effectively. The public is currently advised to eat less and less richly, exercise more and more wisely, avoid undue stress more effectively, self-diagnose and medicate but not inappropriately, smoke less or better still not at all, drink for health's sake but not against health. But this alone will not be enough.

That professional authority, personal effort and public wisdoms all have a part to play in the social construction and management of health care cannot be gainsaid. It is with the sole emphasis on either one of these endeavours or with their unequal financial and moral support that issue is taken. The medical profession has not been notable in promoting health care. Where movement away from a single-minded emphasis on medical treatment is apparent it has been toward *preventive medicine*, a conglomerate of ideals and practices contributory to, but not central, in the active promotion of health. Indeed it would not be too cynical a view that maintains doctors' interest in preventive medicine as a means to counteract escalating costs of treatment and of permitting greater devotion to developments at the frontiers of medical cure in 'interesting cases'. While one would not want to labour the point unduly, the growing support in the present campaign for Health Education among the medical profession does not very obviously suggest any significant change in motive.

Health Care Practice

What then of health care practice? Is the present campaign sufficiently well grounded and oriented? While one would not want to detract one whit from the intention, effort or monies currently devoted to prevention and health, it is not immediately obvious that the enterprise has much to do with the active promotion of health. Notwithstanding the Secretary of State's eagerness to emphasise the rewards of good health as well as the miseries of ill health, it is arguable whether a preventive orientation will provide an adequate basis for health care to flourish.

Indeed we are not as a nation wholly clear as to what health is for. Certainly we have taken some interest latterly in occupational health and more broadly have an expectation of the medical practitioner as a gatekeeper of health to work. But even our occupational health practices are geared to treating disease from industrial hazard and, in some cases, very ambiguously to preventing occupational disease (see Gregory in this volume). It would seem that the thrust is not towards promoting a *healthy* worker, but to procuring the very minimum standards of health which permit full manpower levels to be met. This is so whether in the narrow occupational sense or in a wider sense of general fitness to work.

While it may be a necessary stage toward the development of a genuine National *Health* Service to indulge in the contemporary rhetoric and consciousness raising, one should not mistake the rhetoric for the substance. One should not assume that having provided the words and intention, the necessary substantive changes will ensue.

Health Practitioners

Changes along four dimensions in particular need to be encouraged if the nation is to enjoy an active promotion of health. They are all facets of the development of a more effective health practitioner service. They are, first, more democratic forms of control; second, humane organisation and management systems; third, realistic resource allocation; and finally, changes in inter-professional and professional-client relationships.

These changes may be considered and their achievement initiated within a new ethos concerning the functions and practices of an occupational group which is already trained to work under medical direction in the provision of curative medicine and more particularly charged with providing care to the sick. I refer of course to nurses. Nurses, by reasons of tradition, training and location in the health and medical spheres, within and outside the hospital, are well placed to extend more fully their role toward that of a health care practitioner.

Changes in the nurse's role are not of course unknown. The history of medical advance demonstrates instances where the nurse's role has contracted as new medical specialties developed (e.g. anaesthetics) and where the nurse's role has expanded with new medical discovery (e.g. radium therapy). Indeed the history of nursing care is replete with examples of similar contraction and expansion. When cleanliness and manipulation of the patient's immediate environment constituted the major contribution of care in the cure process only the nurse could be entrusted with it. The greater part of nursing care then was what today would be regarded as non-nursing duties, and nurses have found other avenues of practice (e.g. administration) within which nursing care is demonstrated. Indeed anyone who would venture to redesign the nurse's role must be aware with Gorshenon that 'the role of the nurse is the battle ground for job definition within the health delivery system' (Gorshenon 1970). Yet just because this activity is popular should not deter us from examining the viability and relevance of the nurse as a health practitioner.

I have elsewhere attempted to bring together ideas and arguments in favour of the nurse practitioner and some of the difficulties associated with this extension of role (Austin 1978). There I considered the ways in which health care practice may be enhanced by the development of this ethos, manifest in new types of worker and new locations of nursing work as well as informing nursing knowledge, work arrangements and practices in both more well-known and peripheral locales. One thing is clear. This extension of the nurse's role will be problematic. Problematic because it refers to development of and in an area of enterprise hitherto considered marginal in nursing's usual locales (i.e. the hospital) and work practices (e.g. the health visitor and community nurse on whom there is a work expectation of preventive medicine and promotional health care in relation to certain patient groups). Problematic also because it requires a major conceptual shift to accord to primary health care and its practitioners a discipline, and a moral and financial importance commensurate with that accorded to medical intervention. Problematic too in so far as the development of health care practice severely challenges accepted inter-professional and professional-client relationships. Problematic finally because it requires nurses to find a way through structural obstacles — including those of nursing's own making — to carve out areas of practice knowledge which can be applied to general health care needs.

If health care practice is to be encouraged and if the nurse is to be the major instrument in the development and application of this enhancement of the quality of life, then it is imperative that nursing develop a knowledge-base to underpin the claim of independent practitioner. For *independent* practitioner she must become. To put it in words already quite acceptable when applied to the medical practitioner, she must be a practitioner who exercises clinical judgement within an area of health care expertise which stands alongside, but remains independent of, medical expertise. None of this is to say that nurses will not continue to work in medical locations, nor subordinate some part of their work activities to medical direction. Nursing care beside the doctor's hand and at the patient's bedside will be needed as long as there are diseases and states of ill health amenable to medical treatment and cure. But if a nurse practitioner ethos informs the nurse's 'illness' practices (and is also widely valued) she will be more likely to orient her work to the continuing maintenance of health following the period of medical treatment. In those circumstances, e.g. psychiatric and geriatric conditions where medical cure is inhibited — whether offered within or outside the hospital — the nurse practitioner has more opportunity and scope to encourage the practice of health care to achieve such optimal states of health as medical intervention itself cannot provide, and indeed may negate. Certainly there is no reason why the nurse practitioner – possibly here as a new type of health worker – should not be located in places such as schools, large firms, community agencies, recreation and leisure centres, to develop, promote, maintain and secure health care practices in people *who are not sick.*

Indeed this is the central tenet of the nurse practitioner ethos. The care provided is not to be 'episodic' but 'continual'. Episodic care is periodic and focuses on the patient's illness. Continual care proceeds regardless of whether a person is currently sick. It includes those times, but also carries over to times when the patient has recovered and is alert to preventing other episodes. Allied to the tenet of continual care is that of providing a service beyond the meeting of individual client needs and towards a diagnosis and treatment of community health needs including the range of specialist services required by a given diagnostic group (e.g. maternity, psychiatric) or age group (paediatric, geriatric). There is nothing in the notion of a nurse practitioner which confines her to a medically oriented setting. The locale of her activity fades in importance when set against the work she does. Indeed, this is the main value and importance of the nurse practitioner.

It must be said here that these are not just ideas; examples of these ideas in action are to be found in developed countries such as Canada (Ferguson 1978) and in the activities of the 'barefoot doctors' in developing countries. Indeed it is something of a paradox that, while discussion of the nurse's extended role proceeds in countries spending an appreciable part of their gross national product on medical treatment, the realities of the nurse practitioner's health care activities gathers strength in poorer countries. These countries are either unable, or in some cases self-consciously unwilling (e.g. Tanzania) to devote scarce resources to buy in expensively trained medical personnel to provide high-level skills in a population whose general health profile is thought to need more intermediate intervention including self-help. Of course the social and economic contexts are widely different, but are we sufficiently satisfied with our overall health profiles that we do not also need health practitioners?

Health and Medicine

Of course there is the argument that an enlarged injection of funds would cure the sickness in the NHS. Let us examine this. What it means in effect is that there is a shortage of health service manpower. If there is already a shortage of nurses such that medical intervention cannot proceed with the ease and facility that it would like, what hope is there for the recruitment of new health workers like the nurse practitioner or indeed the diversification of interest towards this ethos among nurses working in the medical sphere?

Some commentators however are not persuaded of the 'overall shortage' argument. They maintain that it is the domination of health service provision by the medical profession that explains the perceived shortage. Leninger's argument, for example, is that dominance by the medical profession primarily oriented toward curing and treating illness stands in the way of even reasonable utilisation of the health care personnel already available (Leninger 1975). Within this counter-argument, it becomes clear that unless this characteristic of current health delivery systems is challenged, then it is not very likely that the encouragement and proliferation of health workers, or the revitalisation of existing health service workers, will do much to alleviate the situation. As a health care system, the NHS has a monolithic structure monopolised by one profession, generally oriented in its education and practice to curing acutely ill, hospitalised persons. This is not solely the result of the self-perception of organised medicine; it is supported by society itself, although increasingly less firmly (Shetland 1975). Health care disciplines, other than medicine, remain relatively unrecognised and unrewarded. Certainly basic primary health care deriving from the sort of general knowledge that is popularly available receives low status in our society. It is either not rewarded at all (see Taylor in this volume) or, in the work world, attracts low prestige and income rewards. Society and medicine's response to the displayed competencies of other health disciplines is to see them as extensions of medicine, encompassed and limited by medical knowledge and ancillary, auxiliary, supplementary or subordinate to medicine.

Evidence of this is the tendency to use health care and medical care interchangeably. However, the concept of health care encompasses preventive measures and refers to the active promotion of health through planning for the maintenance and surveillance of health in communities and families. This is beyond medical competence and requires a range of practice and theoretical knowledge and the talents of several disciplines. These are not usually possessed by practitioners of medicine since they are not formalised within their education and training. If we do not radically reconceptualise our health service provision toward the promotion of health and away from the predominant emphasis on the practice of medicine, any new initiatives in health care practice may extend the medical practitioner's services, but they will not necessarily provide clients with the more varied and appropriate range of services that are widely felt to be needed and deemed lacking.

Many doctors and nurses already subscribe to the view that more direct initiatives should be made in a common pursuit of health. Percipient members of both professions also agree that inter-professional attitudes are out of tune for meeting present health care demands. Such attitudes derive from a patronage system effective in a past era where medical and nursing effort pursued the conquest of environmental and acute disease, but are inappropriate for an ageing population and an increasing incidence of chronic disease and mental illness.

Health Care Organisation

The organisation of health care would be improved if greater efforts were made to address an important issue that underlies the provision of personal service. The issue is about the provision of desired rewards for those whose work is to meet others' personal needs. The question is how best to organise the personal service so that the status needs of practitioners (e.g. income, social standing, community prestige) and the therapeutic needs of clients can be met to their mutual satisfaction. We cannot expect practitioners to go unrewarded; nor can we accept that clients' health needs remain unmet. However, in the current organisation of health service provision neither the status needs of practitioners nor the therapeutic needs of patients seem to be adequately or equitably met.

Nurses have recently sought to satisfy status needs in ways that do not appear to meet the therapeutic needs of clients. I refer to the Salmon reorganisation of the senior nursing structure which gave substantially increased income and status rewards to a newly created hierarchy of nurse administrators (Ministry of Health 1966). It is difficult to determine the extent to which this reorganisation of a significant segment of health service workers serves either the practice of medicine or the promotion of health or indeed the need for status among the *majority* of nurses (Austin 1976).

But it is not difficult to see why the resolution of status needs proceeded in this way and gave rise to the ensuing conflict. Any attempt to add new activities in meeting health and sickness needs proceed with comparative ease when the activities are subordinated to an overarching medical competence. Yet as these new activities are increasingly rewarded so the status of the medical practitioner also increases, based on the claim that he is now doing more skilled work. Thus the status differential remains the same. Conflict arises where non-medical health workers seek parity of status with doctors. For example, where non-medical health workers insist on using knowledge and competencies in responsive and responsible health care decision making in work activities that place them outside the medical sphere. There is no escaping the anxiety and conflict to which this sort of move may give rise. The construction of new roles for health practitioners (a construction not dissimilar to that undertaken by Nightingale and by Salmon, for nurses), drawing on knowledge and competence in a *health* sphere, will involve a part played by medicine; but not necessarily a dominant part. And this realisation needs to be reflected in the future organisation of health care provision.

Recent developments in nursing practice also demonstrate an attempt to democratise health care. With regard to professional-client relationships, nurses are giving more attention to the nursing process — a phrase which connotes the diagnostic skills, implementation and evaluation of nursing — and which is based upon a patient care plan. This plan is seen as a contract between the nurse and the patient which recognises the contribution that patients make toward their own recovery of optimal health. Nursing may have pioneered managerialism in an excessively centralised and closed system model of health care, but it is now patently to be seen as pioneering a recognition of the patient as a factor in the production of the health service.

There is also a growing acknowledgement of a need to construct a health delivery system to which the client can have ready access through a variety of routes. But easier and quicker access will not be enough if what the client meets is a management system devoted solely to efficiency. Personal, and more importantly, personalised service may require the administrators of the health care to put up with less efficient, but no less efficacious, modes of delivery. Indeed one needs to reorganise health care provision to make it more susceptible to citizen input in its development, maintenance and evaluation. Giving Community Health Councils more than the consultative and advisory powers they have at present would be a step in the right direction.

Undoubtedly such an open system will conflict with claims to professional autonomy and clinical freedom. But if we are to behave with regard to our health in the way we are exhorted to behave, then there must be a greater sharing of knowledge between practitioners (doctors and nurses) and clients. Nor is it the case that the corollary of people taking charge of their own health is the abdication of professional authority and professional responsibility. Indeed it is now widely thought that professional responsibility is better served by making professions more accountable to the people and institutions they serve. This does require a diminution of the pervasiveness and rigidity of professional autonomy, but for all that it makes professions no less responsible or authoritative.

It may be argued, for example, that the patient participation achieved in the care plan may alter relationships in the process but leaves the ultimate product untouched. That is, that professional autonomy remains undented because professional authority continues to be imposed. This argument equates authority with autonomy. But while autonomy is claimed on the basis of authority, the claim often goes beyond it. Encouraging patient participation in the process of health care is not only beneficial to the attainment of health, it also re-confines professional autonomy to the limits of professional authority and re-vitalises that authority itself by reminding it of its uncertain base, and its ultimate dependency on patient participation.

A final point about health care organisation is the allocation of resources to the non-hospital sector. If the current campaign of prevention and health is to result in substantive change, then this requires more than just a cosmetic re-allocation of funds to community health practice. It includes recognising the value of the place of practitioners in non-patient agencies and the recruitment and use of volunteer activity in the dissemination of health education and the promotion of health care practice (see Muir and Gray in this volume).

Health Care Roles

Contemporary nursing thought offers a plethora of futures envisaged for the nurse's role. What is evident is that nursing is developing a sense of its multi-dimensional role in the delivery of health care. Health care practice developments within the traditional hospital-doctor setting include highly developed technical skills such as are necessary in intensive care or renal dialysis. At the secondary level of care, nursing is developing clinical expertise in psychiatric and geriatric nursing. Yet another development locates the nursing task at the margin of medical and health care intervention. Here at the primary care level, the nurse would act both as a practising health care worker and as a referral agent to the medical services performing such functions as primary diagnostic screening, routine medical evaluations and counselling.

Yet while nurses are aware of the roles and responsibilities nursing shares with other disciplines it is encouraging to note the increasing awareness that nurses display towards their unique role, one shared with no other discipline.

> It is the role of assisting a patient with his ongoing, minute-by-minute, day-by-day personal care, maintenance, comfort and safety ... very broadly, yet basically stated nursing is a rational and systematic process which deliberately influences the health-illness ecology so as to maximise the possibility of maintaining personal health, safety, comfort and higher levels of wellness for individuals and groups. (Mayers 1973)

This task can remain central just the same, even though nursing develops away from the 'traditional' practice towards concern with the direct and active promotion of health.

The construction of these new roles is, however, not without difficulty. Shetland warns us that within a limited professional training programme, eighteen year old students cannot be expected to acquire a broad and specific set of knowledge and competencies which are probably beyond the attainment of any one human being in a lifetime. Nurses in training are expected to become knowledgeable about nutrition, child guidance, marital and spiritual counselling, physiology, psychology, sociology and in addition to achieve the aims of general education in culture, personal development and good citizenship plus the necessary technical and clinical nursing skills. She concludes by saying 'nursing must learn to limit its claims in terms of reality and reasonable expectations' (Shetland 1975).

But nursing must not only learn to limit its future claims in the proposed new realities, it must also recognise how its present claims are constrained. The medical model is one constraint. Another is that imposed by the bureaucratic structures of hospital or health authority. A system of functional nursing has been the direct consequence of bureaucracy. Functional nursing has resulted in the division of patient care into a series of component tasks performed by different grades of nurse. These grades are organised into a hierarchical control structure which conflicts with the ways nurses are trained to focus on the total care of the patient.

It would be foolish to envisage a wholly non-bureaucratic system of hospital or health care in as large, diverse and complex a society as ours. But it is salutary to note that, on top of the twin subordination of nurses to hospital and health authority bureaucracies, nurses themselves contribute to their own limiting of other nurses via a hierarchical supervisory system which tends to deny professional judgement to the practitioner. These supervision systems, whether professional or bureaucratic, do not permit the practitioner to exercise professional judgement in seeking advice. This is because the actual exercise of such judgement is precisely what is disallowed by the hierarchical structure. If hierarchical systems of control are to remain in the way professions and bureaucracies organise their work, as it seems they must, then the health care professions and bureaucracies must make some effort to ensure that work roles proceed within a clearer knowledge of the areas in which judgement can be exercised and direction must be sought. This recognition of the nurse's freedom to seek advice (as opposed to being directed by supervisor or rule book) is basic to practitioner status and personal service.

The subordination of nurses by nurses is exacerbated by the profession's reliance on nursing procedures. Surprisingly in a profession which has maintained itself as such, nursing is only just beginning to develop a self-conscious knowledge base, which is more than an accumulation of procedures. Procedure-based work activity only becomes intelligible within a subordinated bureaucratic role which does not allow freedom to tailor activity to the person's needs; in short does not permit the display of professional authority. The reaction against nursing procedures as the substance of nursing's professional knowledge (from which authority derives) is demonstrated by a highly commendable search for nursing theory. Some conduct this search within a narrow high science model that looks for a single diagnostic theory; others very laudably emphasise that their enterprise is for theories — and prescriptive ones at that. But what is more important is the insistence with which some search for a development of knowledge which derives from and is rooted in *practice* (e.g. McFarlane 1976). These forms of theorising seek to elaborate the essential work characteristics of nursing viz. caring, helping, assisting, serving towards optimal health, characteristics that I have referred to elsewhere as 'ministering' (Austin 1976).

The ethos of nurse practitioner denotes an emphatic and central concern with nursing practice, with a full development of theories as well as practice, i.e. the delivery of their knowledge and skill. This is most important today. For there is a danger that the learned segment of the health care professions, among them nursing, concerned with more esoteric matters, may leave actual practice out of their deliberations. The development of the nurse practitioner ethos is firmly rooted in practice and so may militate against the bifurcation of the profession into the learned and practising groups. Health care practice deserves no less, and it is clear that the thrust toward independent practitioner status for the nurse in a health care role within a self-conscious *Health* service, must face the structural obstacles set by existing systems of organisation, bureaucracy, profession and knowledge.

Acknowledgements

I am indebted to Marion Ferguson (Lecturer in Nursing at the Department of Advanced Nursing Studies, Welsh National School of Medicine) for discussing many of these ideas with me and for helping me to understand the activity that is nursing.

The substance of this essay was prepared while I was still actively engaged in nursing and health services research. While the ideas and interest remain, the essay must not be taken as anything other than the personal opinion of an officer of the Council for National Academic Awards, the organisation in which I am currently employed. An earlier version of this essay is to be found in *International Nursing Review* Vol. 25 No. 3 1978.

10 A CLINICAL ROLE FOR PHARMACISTS IN THE NHS

Gail Eaton and Barbara Webb

We believe that there is an important role for hospital
pharmacists to play in direct contact with patients on all
matters concerning medication. On the patient's admission,
pharmacists can take the previous medication history; because
of their specialist knowledge they can make an invaluable
contribution in the selection of the drug treatment for the
patient; they can monitor the progress of the medication,
particularly in relation to possible side effects or adverse
reactions; and they can counsel patients on the proper use of
drugs and medicines both in the hospital and when they
return home. (Pharmaceutical Society of Great Britain 1977)

Over the last two decades pharmacists have expressed growing concern
about the nature of their role in the sphere of health care. Traditionally
they have been concerned with the compounding and dispensing of
drugs. However, like a number of other occupations allied to medicine,
they are now seeking to extend their activities into areas previously the
domain of the medical profession.

'Clinical pharmacy', or patient-oriented pharmacy, can be defined as
the application of pharmaceutical knowledge to the clinical situation.
Clinical pharmacists are a segment or group within pharmacy committed
to changing certain aspects of the system of drug use via changes in the
nature of pharmaceutical practice. In defining a new role for
pharmacists they are examining the present system of drug treatment
processes, critically evaluating the knowledge and skill of those personnel at present responsible for drug therapy and identifying gaps and
inadequacies in the system. They suggest that greater use should be
made of the pharmacist, who, through his specialised knowledge of the
pharmaceutical sciences, can provide an expertise in the field of drug
therapy which is lacking in the present system. Clinical pharmacists
seek to intervene at the day-to-day level of patient care where they will
be available to advise both medical practitioner and patient on the
appropriate use of drugs. Rather than just providing the medical practitioner with a pharmaceutical service, ideally the clinical pharmacist is
seen as part of a health care team, all of whose members are equal and

make a unique contribution to patient care.

Clinical Pharmacy in Practice

The Noel Hall Report, which examined the scope and function of the hospital pharmacist, recognised the claims of clinical pharmacists in stating that those with a knowledge of the pharmaceutical sciences could help to promote a safer and more effective use of drugs (DHSS 1970). Many functions outlined in this report were the traditional ones of purchase, quality assurance, quality control, manufacture and distribution. Several of the recommendations, however, called for the pharmacist to extend his role beyond these boundaries. The interpretation and implementation of these functions has become the major part of those evolving activities often referred to as clinical pharmacy.

At a conference in 1977, 34 pharmacists providing clinical services gave details of the schemes organised in their hospitals in the United Kingdom. All those participating had some form of revised drug distribution scheme designed to reduce errors in drug administration. Ward visits were also common, with the purpose of being available to give advice, checking prescriptions for errors and drug interactions and monitoring adverse drug effects. Some pharmacy departments had arranged or were planning to broaden the scope of clinical pharmacy practice into other areas. Just a third of the departments were organising schemes to counsel patients about drug use on admission and discharge. A few had arranged with co-operative consultants for the pharmacist to be present during ward rounds. A drug information service is also being provided in some hospitals; literature is compiled by a pharmacist on drug use and effects and is available to other pharmacists, medical practitioners and nursing staff. Some pharmacy departments act as a repository for reporting on adverse drug reactions and forward such information to the Committee on Safety of Medicines. Two departments were planning to set up 'consultant' pharmacy posts; others proposed or actually attended clinical meetings with medical practitioners. Still others carried out laboratory tests to establish drug levels in body fluids and some were involved in research (Hospital Group of the Pharmaceutical Society of Great Britain 1977).

There have been a number of studies reported in this country, but more particularly in the United States, demonstrating that clinical pharmacy schemes reduce prescribing errors and encourage more appropriate prescribing, thereby contributing to better patient care. One recent study claimed that 61 per cent of all drug treatment was irrational in the pharmacist's estimation – 18 per cent being deemed serious enough to warrant communication with the prescribing physician (Vance 1973).

The significance of clinical pharmacy schemes is principally that pharmacists have taken it upon themselves to examine errors in drug administration and to evaluate the performance of those making decisions about drug therapy. The motives and interests of pharmacists who are involved in such schemes are clear: to demonstrate the need for some kind of safety check and to indicate that the intervention of some suitably qualified expert, more specifically a clinical pharmacist, is necessary.

The attempts by pharmacists to expand their role to encompass a clinical dimension are not new: Poston (personal communication) has documented the aspirations of pharmacists in this sphere as described in the pharmaceutical literature at the beginning of the twentieth century. And, of course, even prior to this century, their direct access to patients in the community has involved chemists and druggists in giving medical advice unofficially − colloquially their premises were known as 'doctors' shops' in the last century amongst that section of the population who had no means of access to the formal medical care provided by physicians.

The apothecaries were the traditional compounders and dispensers of drugs, although by the nineteenth century they had largely forsaken this role in favour of medical practice. With the establishment of a Medical Register by Act of Parliament in 1858, these 'general practitioners' were incorporated into the ranks of the esteemed medical profession alongside those who held the title 'physician' and 'surgeon'. Chemists and druggists came to be principally responsible for the compounding and dispensing of medicines from retail premises. This group, anticipating their exclusion from the Medical Register, had established their own occupational association, the Pharmaceutical Society, in 1841. The association's stated aims were 'to benefit the public and elevate the profession of Pharmacy, by furnishing the means of proper instruction to protect the collective and individual interests and privileges of all its members, in the event of any hostile attack in Parliament or otherwise' (Bell and Redwood 1880).

Chemists and druggists, or 'pharmacists', as they came to be known, deliberately chose to disassociate themselves from the tasks of medical practitioners as illustrated by the following extract from the Pharmaceutical Journal of 1845. 'We look forward to the time when it will be considered as much beneath the dignity of a Pharmaceutical Chemist to become an irregular Medical Practitioner, as it would be derogatory to a

Physician to practise Pharmacy' (Crellin 1967).

The pharmacists aimed to establish their work upon a scientific basis although the apprenticeship system of training persisted until the late 1960s when universal graduate entry was achieved. But by this time practising pharmacists had lost their traditional compounding role to the pharmaceutical industry and many of their skills acquired during a lengthy university course were proving redundant in practice. Furthermore pharmacists had failed to achieve a monopoly over the one area of work – dispensing – which could be said to be a truly pharmaceutical activity. Medical practitioners have retained the right to dispense their own medicines, although in their evidence to the Royal Commission pharmacists take the opportunity to emphasise the limits they would like to set to general practitioner dispensing. 'To support the principle that physicians should prescribe and pharmacists should dispense, dispensing by medical practitioners should be limited to those rural areas where the public would otherwise experience serious difficulty in having prescriptions dispensed by a pharmacist.' And as the government has permitted other retail outlets apart from pharmacies to sell non-prescribed medicines, pharmacists have also failed in their efforts to convince those in power that these substances are a special commodity whose sale requires the supervision of someone skilled in pharmaceutics.

Clinical pharmacy can be described as a 'professionalising mcvement' within pharmacy. Appeals have been made to the unconverted amongst pharmacists, that the occupation as a whole would enjoy enhanced status in its relations with the public and the medical profession by the adoption of a clinical approach to pharmacy practice. In recently published literature it has been claimed that 'the rewards of professionalisation outweigh its obligations' (Smith and Knapp 1972), and that 'pharmacy is called to a higher level' (McGlothlin 1964). Attempts have also been made to persuade the government, the medical profession and the public that the promotion of a clinical orientation to pharmacy practice will result in higher standards of drug prescribing by medical practitioners, better utilisation of drugs by patients, and a decrease in the cost of prescribed medicines to the nation.

However, there are problems for clinical pharmacists in achieving their aims. One problem is that education in the past has not been concerned to prepare pharmacists for any kind of clinical involvement. Consequently, clinical pharmacists have made energetic attempts to influence academic pharmacists. It was apparent to us in the course of a research project on the aims and current objectives of educational pharmacists, that all were aware of the changes taking place in hospital practice, and those who were in agreement with this orientation had incorporated into the pharmacy syllabus subjects which were basic to the medical school curriculum, e.g. pathology and the aetiology of disease. In some instances, visits to hospital wards were arranged for those students who took a 'clinical pharmacy option', and there was talk of organising certain lectures jointly with medical students where a good relationship existed between the medical and pharmacy schools. A reorientation of this kind, it was felt, would give the qualified pharmacist a better understanding of the relationship between diagnosis and treatment and allow him to communicate more effectively with the prescribing physician. This had been identified as one of the principal problems in relations between medical practitioners and pharmacists in the past.

Clinical Pharmacy and the Medical Profession

Concern at problems of drug use has not been limited to pharmacists. The publicity given to the thalidomide tragedy led to increased public awareness of the problems of adverse drug effects. Within the medical profession, certain individuals were becoming interested in these problems and recognising that medical practitioners themselves often had insufficient knowledge of the actions and effects of powerful modern drugs. Clinical pharmacology was the name given to describe this area of study. Its development as a medical specialty was given added impetus by the continuing identification of drug problems during the subsequent decade. Clinical pharmacologists aim 'to promote safer and more effective prescribing', and they define their subject matter as 'the scientific study of how drugs affect the body and how the body affects drugs'. They claim that knowledge of the actions and effects of drugs in the patient has not kept pace with the growth of the pharmaceutical industry's production of drug preparations. They also argue that in the past insufficient attention has been paid to teaching medical students about the therapeutic use of drugs during their training. Postgraduate education does not appear to compensate for this; indeed the extent of drug company involvement in post-graduate education has been a further subject of adverse criticism.

Clinical pharmacologists, not unnaturally, have been the group within medicine most interested in the claims made by the proponents of clinical pharmacy. Almost all those clinical pharmacologists we interviewed in the course of our research perceived the pharmacist as having a valuable contribution to make at the ward level. Most felt that while there was a place for the pharmacist in the 'health care team' this should be confined to giving advice on the formulation, strength and dosage of drugs. They did not consider it appropriate for pharmacists to have any greater role in treatment decisions on the grounds that they possessed insufficient knowledge of diagnosis. It is clear that the justification for clinical pharmacology rests primarily upon the assumption that certain essential contributions can only be made by persons who are medically qualified. This is illustrated in the unpublished evidence given by clinical pharmacologists to the Royal Commission on the NHS:

> Rational drug usage represents a complicated interplay between the patient's disease and the contribution that drug therapy (when properly applied) can offer in its alleviation. For this reason, drug prescribing cannot be divorced from other aspects of patient management. And since the management of a patient is the responsibility of his medical attendant, we are opposed to any system whereby drug prescribing is devolved to others except under special circumstances. Neither registered nurses, *nor qualified pharmacists, are competent to initiate or regulate drug therapy.* Clinical supervision is essential [our italics].

The response of the Chairman of the BMA General Medical Services Committee to the 'clinical' aspirations of certain pharmacists was a little less diplomatic:

> I don't think the pharmacist needs a stronger role: the pharmacist's role should be clearly identified and if they concentrated on that and spent less time on toilet paper and soaps and things, then perhaps it might be to the advantage of their profession. (*Pharmaceutical Journal* 5 February 1977)

In practice there is no obvious conflict between clinical pharmacists and clinical pharmacologists; both groups are small in number and at the present time they do not frequently confront each other in work settings. Clinical pharmacologists are mainly confined to the teaching hospitals and have tended to direct their efforts towards improving the drug knowledge of their fellow physicians at the educational level. Clinical pharmacists, on the other hand, are attempting to influence drug use on the wards and few ever encounter a clinical pharmacologist in their daily work.

Increasingly, however, there is greater contact between clinical pharmacologists and clinical pharmacists. The former have sought to expand their activities into district general hospitals and where clinical pharmacologists have been employed in this capacity they have taken over the organisation of activities such as the provision of drug information services and the monitoring of drug interactions and adverse effects. The pharmacist may still be involved, but the medically qualified clinical pharmacologist is responsible for the 'clinically relevant' aspects of the work. The clinical pharmacologist, it is claimed, is better able to advise other medical practitioners.

Pharmacists have in fact challenged the need for a clinical pharmacologist in the district general hospital on the basis that it is illogical to introduce this when there are existing personnel in the hospital (pharmacists) competent to carry out the functions which clinical pharmacologists have identified as being within the realm of medical practice.

Boundary Encroachment and Defence

Pharmacy is one of the occupations which has been termed paramedical in that its central tasks are organised around those of medicine, the dominant profession. Within the NHS, the tasks of pharmacists have traditionally been carried out on the instructions of medical practitioners, the dispensing of drugs is requested once a diagnosis and treatment decision has been reached by the physician. Pharmacists are only one group among the many occupations supplementary to medicine (physiotherapists, dieticians, radiographers are others) who have been concerned in recent years to re-evaluate their relationship with the medical profession and to redefine their role in the health care sphere. Recently it has been argued that the expansionist designs and activities of such paramedical groups indicate that these occupations are increasing their power and status at the expense of the medical profession. It is claimed the medical profession's position of pre-eminence has been severely weakened as a result of this.

We would argue from our own study of the clinical pharmacy movement, that there is little evidence to support this view. It is clear that pharmacists who are engaged in 'clinical activities' are concerned not to appear to challenge the physician's authority. In our interviews it was stressed continually that in order to be 'accepted' by physicians, the clinical pharmacist must employ strategies of tact and diplomacy. The aim is to persuade the medical practitioner to utilise the skills the pharmacist has to offer by conciliatory measures. And it is significant that the medical practitioner is usually required to take the initiative in availing himself of the proffered service. Those engaged in clinical pharmacy schemes speak of 'providing advice to physicians when this is solicited'. In this way medical practitioners retain the right to decide whether or not to seek the pharmacists' advice and service, and the success or failure of clinical pharmacy schemes often depends upon co-operation – or lack of it – from the medical profession. Under no circumstances is the pharmacist, acting in his advisory capacity, to adopt the physician's role in diagnosing illness and prescribing treatment. The retail pharmacist in dealing directly with the public's minor health problems, does not, it is claimed, diagnose or prescribe; he is rather engaging in a process of 'differential diagnosis', that is, helping the public to distinguish between conditions that can be self-treated and those that should be referred to a physician. This linguistic caution reflects the concern of pharmacists not to usurp the role of the physican nor to challenge his clinical freedom

Again it was frequently reiterated in our interviews that the ideal situation is one where the physician will utilise the skills of the pharmacist as to the choice of drug, its form and dosage, when both are members of the same team. The concept of teamwork is one much favoured by paramedical occupations. Yet pharmacists themselves, whilst advocating a teamwork approach to treatment none the less accept implicitly that within a team of co-operating health care professions, those medically qualified must retain the leadership role.

> We should be considered as members of a team and the boundaries, the duties should depend more upon the particular attributes of the individual than upon academic convenience . . . [but] the consultant physician must be the leader of this team, . . . he must take overall responsibility. (Head of Pharmacy School)

It would appear that pharmacists are lending support to the arguments used by clinical pharmacologists in their evidence to the Royal Commission.

The way in which the medical profession has accommodated the activities of clinical pharmacists can be seen as an instance of task delegation. The medical profession has traditionally delegated certain tasks to those in paramedical occupations. Hospital nurses, for example, sometimes take the decision to 'prescribe' certain drugs, in particular sedatives and analgesics, when they deem this necessary. In general practice it is common for receptionists to issue repeat prescriptions and advise patients on the treatment of minor ailments. Although medical practitioners often will not admit to or condone such practices, they are willing to 'turn a blind eye' to them, and in this way activities which began merely as convenient 'short-cuts' in work routines have now become areas of informal task delegation. Such delegation does not detract from the status and authority of the medically qualified who remain, theoretically at least, ultimately responsible for the patient. And it is clinical responsibility which gives the medical profession status and authority in its dealings with patients and other paramedical groups.

Those activities in which pharmacists have shown interest, are in areas where medical practitioners have taken the kinds of 'short-cuts' described above or which they have neglected — for example patient counselling on drug use, monitoring of drug side effects and the provision of drug information services. By the assumption of such tasks the pharmacist may gain in status *vis-à-vis* other paramedical workers, he may even gain the medical practitioner's tacit affirmation that he is better equipped to make decisions about drugs than the hospital nurse or the general practice receptionist, but this will not fundamentally affect the relative positions of pharmacy and medicine in the occupational hierarchy.

While the status quo remains unaltered, the notion that a revised pharmacy school curriculum will effect major changes in practice may prove ill founded. The graduate pharmacist may find that his employment in a provincial hospital with limited activities on the ward does not permit the utilisation of his newly acquired knowledge and skill. One British Professor of Pharmacy, visiting a clinical pharmacy scheme in the United States, illustrated these kinds of problems in the following account:

I heard them saying pharmacists should give injections and I asked why. Well, I was told, nurses are in short supply. So then I got to see the clinical pharmacist on the ward and I asked: 'Are you in charge of this floor?' Yes. 'You are a clinical pharmacist?' Yes. 'Tell me what your function is.' Well, I'm sort of in charge of this floor. 'Yes, but what do you do?' Well, I go around with the doctors and see things. 'Yes, but what do you do?' Well if there is an interaction, I bring it to his attention. 'Suppose the doctor tells you to get lost, what do you do?' Oh well — he's in charge isn't he.

It cannot be denied that many of the problems which have been identified as arising from current practice in drug prescribing can be greatly reduced. What remains to be asked is whether pharmacists are the best or only people suited to effect such improvements. Could nursing and medical staff carry out these tasks just as effectively if this were demanded of them? Moreover, can the NHS withstand the cost of providing clinical pharmacists to cover every ward in every hospital, as well as those pharmacists who remain to perform technical and dispensing functions? It is worth noting here that the Aberdeen drug distribution scheme, the first of its kind instigated by a pharmacist which served as a protocol for others all over the country, is becoming increasingly difficult to operate due to lack of finance.

It could be argued that pharmacists have played their most significant role in pointing out the location of certain weaknesses in the present system of drug treatment and showing how these can be remedied. Economic considerations, combined with the awareness within the medical profession that there is a need to 'put its own house in order' and doing this in such a way as to preserve the special status of clinicians, may prevent the clinical pharmacist from assuming any greater role in patient care.

The Pharmacist and Patient Care

The principal claim of pharmacists advocating a 'clinical' pharmacy has been that patients will benefit from the resulting improvements in the standards of drug treatment. Given that this is a constantly recurring theme, do such schemes fundamentally affect the well-being of patients in the NHS?

It has been claimed that retail pharmacists have long played a 'clinical' role, largely unacknowledged and without being graced with such a title. The activities of the retail pharmacist have traditionally included advising customers on self-medication. And it is claimed that in dispensing medicines prescribed by medical practitioners, pharmacists are automatically involved in clarifying instructions with the patient and medical practitioner and checking for errors. Several studies have provided evidence of the valuable contribution made by the pharmacist to primary health care, advising those with minor symptoms on their self-care and referring those with potentially serious symptoms to their general practitioner.

Included in the Pharmaceutical Society's evidence to the Royal Commission are proposals that the retail pharmacists' ability to give advice on the treatment of 'minor ailments' be recognised, and that pharmacists should be able to 'prescribe' certain drugs at present reserved for prescription only. And indeed much of the present public and governmental concern about the increase in the number of retail pharmacy closures in recent years centres upon the perceived loss to the community of such a service.

However, there have also been a few studies which have attempted to evaluate critically the service to the patient provided by the retail pharmacist. One study in the United States examined the extent to which pharmacists advised the patient on the use of non-prescribed medicines (Wertheimer and Smith 1974). A research assistant posing as a diabetic discussed his condition with a pharmacist and then proceeded to purchase an over-the-counter preparation contra-indicated for use by diabetics. Eighty-three per cent of pharmacists either sold the product or recommended another often more expensive brand, also contra-indicated for use by diabetics. A survey of 183 British pharmacies by the Consumers' Association in 1975 produced findings which gave similar cause for concern. When a researcher described symptoms of a potentially serious nature, one pharmacist in five failed to give advice or sold unhelpful or inappropriate medicine, and only about half the pharmacists mentioned seeing a doctor.

Certainly the fact that the retail pharmacist operates a business may result in his commercial interests conflicting with his professional discretion. Or it may simply be that for those pharmacists who have no inclination to play a 'patient-oriented role' there is little incentive, financial or otherwise, to do so. And there is another constraint which limits the retail pharmacist's involvement in patient care. If the pharmacist has reason to question the appropriateness of a prescription and takes the trouble to raise the matter with the medical practitioner, the latter is in no way obliged to take the pharmacist's advice. Cases where the prescribing physician acts in this way may be rare, but they nevertheless indicate a major loophole in the argument that the pharmacist acts as a 'safety-valve'. The pharmacist's role as adviser to both patient and prescribing physician is thus severely limited by such factors.

In hospital pharmacy the problems arising from the commercialism of retail pharmacy do not apply, but constraints deriving from the nature of the relations between pharmacist and physician still operate. In one ward pharmacy scheme that we were acquainted with the ward pharmacist was careful not to be present during the consultant's ward rounds because it was felt that the latter might find it difficult to 'take advice' from the pharmacist. Instead, the pharmacist would do his own 'ward round' reporting back if necessary to the physician. Intrusion into spheres is thus effected in a way likely to cause as little offence as possible to the medical profession.

It is arguable that the solution pharmacists have proposed to problems in drug treatment, whilst doubtless effecting some improvement in patient care, may none the less create other problems. Pharmacists do not appear to have considered that, in assuming a more active role drug treatment which allows them to act in a more recognisably 'professional' capacity, they may make similar errors and be responsible for similar gaps and inadequacies in the system. It is taken for granted that professional standards safeguard the patient and assumed that such standards guarantee a high level of competency. The criticisms levelled at the medical profession are assumed to be due to the deficiencies of those medically qualified. Problems which could be said to arise from the nature of professional-client relations in the health service, such as difficulties in communication between patients and medical personnel, have been neglected by pharmacists. There appears to be no consideration in the literature written by clinically involved pharmacists of the increased role that the consumer might play in his own drug treatment. Nor is any attention given to the fact that the addition of another 'professional' may further increase the existing problems in communication for the patient.

Consumer critics of the health service have asked if patients' needs and interests should always be defined by professionals and whether colleague control really is a sufficient safeguard for the patient. Such criticisms of professional behaviour apply equally to those occupations like pharmacy seeking to become 'more professional'. The consumer may be forgiven for asking whether intra-occupational conflict and bargaining for power, status and responsibility, have any bearing upon the problems they perceive to exist in the health service. Physicians have been criticised by consumers for being too drug-oriented in their approach to treatment; pharmacists' involvement in treatment processes and decision making, with their minimal knowledge of therapeutics (i.e. treatment as a whole, not merely drug treatment), is not likely to redress this bias.

It presents something of a contradiction for pharmacists to criticise physicians' prescribing on the one hand, whilst upholding clinical autonomy – the right of the physician to prescribe what he chooses – on the other. This is further reflected in pharmacists' demands to play a more active role in drug therapy, preferably as a member of a team, whilst conceding that the physician must retain the position as 'leader'. Again, pharmacists want more responsibility for patient care, yet admit that ultimate responsibility for the patient must lie with the medical practitioner. These dilemmas have not, as yet, been satisfactorily resolved. Pharmacists have been critical without seeming to challenge the medical mandate, and this is surely because if pharmacists are too critical of the medical profession they will not gain the goodwill and co-operation upon which clinical pharmacy schemes are reliant.

Acknowledgements

In preparing this paper we have drawn on unpublished research conducted during 1975-78, funded by the Department of Health and Social Security, examining the development and present organisation of clinical pharmacy and clinical pharmacologists. We have quoted interviews with heads of schools of pharmacy and clinical pharmacologists.

PORTERS' PROBLEMS, DOCTORS' DILEMMAS

John Grigg

If journalists evinced any real interest in industrial *relations* as opposed
to industrial conflict one might have seen headlines in the national
dailies in 1968 celebrating 'Twenty Years of Industrial Peace in the
NHS'. While that headline remained merely unlikely a decade ago it
would be an impossibility today, because industrial conflict has now
become a marked feature of the health service. Since 1970, and more
noticeably since 1972, journalists have been able to indulge their
penchant for reducing industrial relations to stories about strikes by
documenting concerted industrial action by porters, cooks, domestics,
pathology laboratory technicians, radiographers, nurses, junior hospital
doctors and consultants. This enormous increase in strike activity has
been matched by an increase in what health service managers describe as
union militancy and, an associated phenomenon, the acquisition of an
industrial relations vocabulary. The DHSS commissioned Lord
McCarthy to enquire into the workings of the Whitley Council structure
and is now sponsoring high-level skills training for an emergent group of
industrial relations managers within the health service. Yet the whole
area of industrial relations in the NHS is but sketchily mapped.

In this short chapter I propose quite slavishly to follow the journal-
istic trend and to concentrate on a subsidiary theme of strikes, the
notion of cost involved in taking industrial action, by looking at aspects
of industrial action taken by two groups of health service staff, ancillary
workers and doctors.

Both these groups of staff have resorted to strike action or to
working to rule within the last six years. Yet there the similarities
would seem to end. It would be hard to think of two more different
groups of NHS staff, ranged at opposite ends of almost any axes one
can think of. Yet, despite these massive differences in class, occupation
structure, occupational control, pay, status within the hospital and so
on, I will argue that there are critical similarities between doctors and
ancillary workers *when they resort to industrial action*. I will suggest
that the socially sensitive nature of their occupations and the palpable
and visible immediacy of the social consequences of their industrial
actions constrain both groups of workers to manage those actions in
quite similar ways.

The notion of cost in the analysis of collective bargaining has received its most brilliant exposition in the work of Walton and McKersie (1965). During any industrial action the parties to that action are engaged in a constant process of evaluation of the costs involved. These costs may be material, ideological, or personal. Thus the opponents in the conflict will attempt, consciously or unconsciously, to cost out the implications of taking or resisting certain actions, and this costing process will help determine strategy, tactics, and the outcome of the negotiations. In the course of a strike in, say, the production industry (or indeed in any enterprise substantially dominated by the profit motive) it is likely that the major calculations will all centre on the material costs. If, for example, the Dagenham plant of Fords is on strike then, explicitly or implicitly, workers and management engage in costing the impact of the strike on production, orders, loss of sales revenue; in short to profits. Of course, costing is not, and cannot be, confined to money. Lane (1972), Beynon (1974) and Hyman (1972) all point to the many other calculations which take place. Yet money is a convenient focus for disparate grievances, so the financial calculation is the one which receives the greatest publicity.

An early stage in a dispute is distinguished by emphasis on cost. Each side points to the costs borne by the other of maintaining its position.

> . . . thus the union will try to convince management that refusal to adjust its position will certainly result in a strike, and the union will emphasise the costs of the strike to the company. The employer's equivalent tactic is to emphasise the damage resulting from acceptance of the union's target: that it will bankrupt the company or the whole national economy and the union members will be unemployed. (Anthony and Crichton 1969:111)

I take this to mean that one side says 'if you insist on doing that we will ensure that it is going to cost you a lot'. The other side also says 'if you don't stop this useless resistance it will cost you even more'. So, to take our simple example, the Ford workers promise that it will cost Ford's management much more in lost profits than it would cost them to meet the workers' wage demands. Characteristically then, the strikers *stress* the impact of their sanctions on the continued well-being of the enterprise, and in particular on the profits of that enterprise.

In their turn the managers will assess not only the effects the sanctions will have, on profits, on intangibles such as the sanctity of grievance procedures, on managerial prerogatives and on the saving accruing on not having to pay wages to the strikers, but also on the workers' capacity to 'stand the strike'. That is, the management will attempt to evaluate the strength of feeling behind the action and the ability of the unions to pay strike-pay. Perhaps the most vivid illustration of the *reflexive* effect of taking strike action is contained in those descriptions of lines of gaunt colliers gradually starving rather than giving in to the pit owners, the common currency of historical novels of nineteenth-century working-class life. The second aspect of the 'reflexive' costing will be the consideration by the strikers themselves of the costs to them of taking action. Once again it must be emphasised that these costs will not always, or even usually, be financial costs. A frequently documented aspect of the alleged irrationality of strikers' behaviour is that where a crude balance sheet is drawn up making invidious comparisons between the wages lost by workers during a protracted strike and the (usually lesser) sums extracted from management by the strike action. As Hyman (1972) notes, such apparently self-damaging and irrational behaviour seems much more sensible and rational when viewed from a perspective which takes account of man's attachment to principles rather than profit. So an important element of the reflexive cost then must be the impact of industrial action on union growth and notions such as 'workers' rights', 'solidarity' and 'defiance'; in short, the meanings of the action for the actors.

When we apply this analysis to groups taking industrial action within the National Health Service, we are forced to consider the peculiar nature of public employment in a service area involving public safety (*pace* the firemen, possibly the most sensitive service area involved in public safety). That is, we have to look at the limitations which are inevitably imposed on those who take industrial action which disrupts the provision of the service and whose actions are potentially or actually threatening life in the most direct way. The socially sensitive position of the NHS or any other health service does not need illustration; if the service is withdrawn, people die. If the consequences of industrial action are (or can be made to seem) of such critical immediacy and significance, then the notion of the cost of sanctions in this area is thrown into high relief.

The most obvious initial problem facing the striker in the National Health Service is the difficulty of forcing the employer to see the strike as costing money. One of the interesting features of the protracted ancillary workers' strike of 1972/3 was the virtual abdication of interest by Hospital Management Committees and Regional Hospital Boards in the progress of the strike; they were, in Winkler's evocative phrase, 'ghosts at the bargaining table'. Indeed, in some cases, they were even jovial ghosts. One Regional Hospital Board Treasurer informed me that the strike was saving him money because he did not have to pay the strikers. In the absence of a profit motive to strike at the health service workers are faced with a paradox. That is, to convince the management of the seriousness of their intentions they should, as we have seen, maximise the impact of their actions on the service. Yet to emphasise the effectiveness of sanctions by pointing to the only obvious (though problematic) consequences of their actions, namely deaths or worsening illnesses for the patients, could not be a recommended course of action. Nor was such an emphasis attempted, either by the ancillary workers or the doctors.

If we look at the tactics of the ancillary workers during their action in the winter of 1973 the paradox can be illustrated by the opening statement made by the central co-ordinating committee of the four major unions involved (National Union of Public Employees, Confederation of Health Service Employees, Transport and General Workers Union and the General and Municipal Workers Union). The statement said that the co-ordinating committee's 'aim is not to cause hardship or suffering for patients. Members will continue to operate essential services, such as operating theatres, for emergency cases'. Although the union leaders conceded that their aim was to force hospitals to cut back or abandon routine medicine they attempted to stress that their sanctions would harm no one.

In the same way both the consultants, who began a work-to-contract in December 1975, and the junior hospital doctors, whose industrial conflict with the DHSS was proceeding at the same time, felt constrained to point out that no harm was going to come to the patients as a result of their actions. In all three cases these optimistic statements were actively challenged in the press and on television and radio, and in all three cases much of the critical public management of the industrial action centred on the notion of the 'emergency'. There is, of course, no firm distinction between the 'non-acute' and the 'acute' case. Clinical definitions of acute need are in many important respects social definitions, so what constitutes an 'emergency' in one clinician's judgement may not be so defined in another's. Nor is the definition imposed unilaterally, despite the medical profession's greater power to label. It is a negotiated process. In some cases ancillary worker pickets attempted to challenge clinical definitions of emergencies at the hospital gates, and there is evidence that, throughout the ancillary workers' action, much of the local level bargaining between them and the management centred on the distinctions between 'acute' and 'non-acute' admissions.

In the ordinary way of things it can be contended that public relations has very little to do with the outcome of any particular strike. Industrial relations is about power. If the nation needs coal and the miners refuse to dig it then the issue is essentially a very simple one, and no amount of publicity about old-age pensioners dying of hypothermia is likely to make significant impact on the outcome of that strike. And anyway, it is an accepted common tactic of the NUM and other unions involved in similar actions to make sure that the social impact of their actions is limited. Thus, they aim for publicity showing miners taking their own coal to old-age pensioners to ensure that the latter do not suffer as a result of the major action. Similarly the power workers can be seen to be active in ensuring that places like hospitals are kept working even when the rest of us are plunged into darkness. In the case of the National Health Service, and indeed with the public sector generally, it can be contended that the impact of public relations is much more significant. Thus ancillary workers and doctors alike made great efforts to ensure that their case was presented sympathetically to the public; much play was made with the idea that their sanctions were aimed at 'cold' medicine and that the safety of the general public was guaranteed simply by arrangements made for emergency cover.

The public debate was thereby simplified into crudely opposing definitions of safety and harm. 'Cold' medicine could be interfered with, even brought to a stop, but no lasting harm to the public would result. If satisfactory arrangements could be made to deal with medical emergencies then all would be well. It is in this area that we see some very interesting manipulations of the definitions of well-being and harm by the medical profession in particular. For example, in early March 1973, after porters, cleaners, laundry workers and catering staff had been on (partial) strike for less than two weeks, a statement signed by the Chairman of Birmingham's five Medical Executive Committees, and claiming to represent some 300 consultants employed by the (then) Birmingham Regional Hospital Board, stated that 'some patients will suffer permanent ill health, disability and for some people, death at an earlier date than would have been the case had our normal hospital services been available' (*Guardian* report 13 March 1973). Similar statements crowded the letter columns of *The Times* newspaper throughout the dispute. Yet when the consultants themselves were working to contract almost two years later one could search the press and the letter columns in vain for equivalent statements from those same Birmingham consultants. Indeed, the strike leaders of the junior hospital doctors and the consultants issued press releases remarkably like those made by the ancillary workers' unions in March and April 1973.

This active condemnation of the effects of two weeks of *partial* strike action by ancillary workers and the soothing reassurances about the impact of similar action by the medical profession itself rather draws one to the conclusion that the presence of ancillary workers in hospitals is essential to the health of the patients, the absence of doctors merely an inconvenience. However, I do not wish to overstate the case. Both *The Lancet* (27 December 1975) and the *BMJ* (22 November 1975) carried editorials during the industrial action by the juniors and the consultants which presented the difficulties facing the profession very clearly.

The junior hospital doctors have a reasonable cause for grievance – the Consultants have a much stronger case – but patients are suffering and will certainly die as a result of industrial action by any member of the health service, be they porters, nurses or doctors. We have no quarrel with our patients, and refusing to treat them when they are ill is no different from terrorists endangering innocent lives, believing their cause a just one. Please – all in the NHS – don't forget the patient (*BMJ* 22 November 1975).

Similarly in *The Lancet* on 27 December 1975, 'at no time during these latest troubles in the NHS have any doctors had even remotely acceptable reasons for withdrawing their best efforts from some of their patients – whether what the doctors did was in the name of professional freedom or in the furtherance of a play claim'.

'We would apply these strictures unreservedly, even to the threat of mass resignations from the NHS, which in the absence of an alternative service other than the medical market place, is industrial action by another name.' Both these quotations are printed in Iliffe and Gordon's *Pickets in White* (1977). However, the authors of this pamphlet fail to take up the argument. Instead they say:

they i.e. the views of the *BMJ* and *The Lancet* leader writers can certainly not be dismissed as unrealistic views, although both essentially fail to grasp the point. There is no inherent contradiction between the professional responsibility of a doctor, his contribution to society's needs and his being paid according to the work he actually does.

This does not seem to answer the point made by the two journals. The editorials stress the incompatibility of the notion of 'professional' with action which endangers patients. *Pickets in White* glosses over this. However, Iliffe and Gordon do point to the significance of the united condemnation of the press of the doctors' actions. There were, it will be remembered, some particularly harrowing cases widely publicised, including the case of a baby girl who died after being ferried by ambulance from hospital to hospital, allegedly being unable to receive treatment at the accident and emergency departments of two of them.

Generally union leaders of the ancillary workers attempted to avoid discussions about the ultimate effects of their action and instead concentrated on the rather less central difficulties which were presented to patients accommodated in the hospitals where the domestic staff refused to wash up and the laundry staff refused to launder the hospital linen. For example, the Deputy South Wales Divisional Officer of NUPE, Mr Edward Elms, said that 'despite the disposable plates the patients will not even know the difference' (*Western Mail*, 2 March 1973). In addition it is noteworthy that the unions generally readily agreed to widespread use of volunteer labour or the intervention of other health service staff in their jobs — 'Medical staffs become maids of all work' headline in *The Times*, 2 March 1973. This is interesting because it means that the unions involved effectively prevented the pursuit of those very tactics which they hoped would bring about a speedy and, to them, satisfactory resolution of their conflict. By importing volunteer workers, which in any other industrial situation would have been importing 'black-legs', the strikers connived at their own strike breaking. Indeed, in some cases the effect of the paradox forced them to go further than this. There are well-documented instances of strikers black-legging *themselves.* For example, on 6 March the *Western Mail* reported that South Wales' Secretary to the Strike Co-ordinating Committee, Mr Norman Waring, had said 'it is in the laundry workers' best interests to provide some sort of emergency service on a volunteer basis'.

It must not be assumed that these Health Service strikers were forced into these and other self-contradictory actions *simply* by the féar that their tactics would alienate public sympathy. At the risk of stressing the obvious, the difference is this: striking miners have no attachment to coal *as* coal, nor do they go home and worry about the amount of coal that they have not dug while they are striking. But doctors and porters are all human beings, claiming to have an essentially humane and compassionate concern for the sick which is, in the case of the doctors, formally codified in such ritual pronouncements as the Hippocratic oath. Sanctions which strike at the well-being of patients strike at one of the central ideological pillars of professionalism and at a central humanity which we all share. That is, most of us think it wrong to let people die. It is precisely for these reasons that the reflexive effect of exerting sanctions has such a powerful impact on the would-be strikers. This is not the place for an extended discussion on the ethics of causing death and saving lives (see Glover 1977). However, professionalism and some kind of ethic of service to the patient are closely interlinked.

The early sociological literature on professionalism has been described by Johnson (1972) as falling into two main streams and adopting two similar models to describe the phenomenon, which he terms the 'trait' model and the 'functionalist' model. In the 'trait' model writers such as Carr-Saunders and Wilson (1933) and Millerson (1964) attempted to list the characteristics of existing professions; for example, adherence to a code of conduct, the possession of skill based on theoretical knowledge, provision of training and education and testing the competence of members, and an ethic of service to the community.

Those theorists Johnson calls the 'functionalists' proceeded in a rather similar fashion except that they consider only those elements of the profession's characteristic traits thought to make a functional contribution to the relationship between professional and client or to the maintenance of society. Thus Barber describes, among other things, the following:

> essential attributes of professionalism . . . a primary orientation to the community interests rather than individual self-interest; a high degree of self-control of behaviour through codes of ethics internalised in the process of work socialisation organised and operated by the work specialists; and a system of rewards (monetary and honorary) that is primarily a set of symbols of work achievement and thus ends in themselves, not means to some end of individual self-interest (Barber 1963).

Later, Paul Halmos claimed that 'a service ethic' characterised professional organisation; of course he specifically singled out medicine as one such profession (Halmos 1970). In all cases, then, a common element in descriptions of professions has been that they profess to serve the public, to place their own personal interests behind those of the client or patient, and even to 'give the consumer not what he wants (however profitable) but what he needs' (Klein 1973).

It is much more difficult to point to a similar scholarly buttressing for my next contention, but I still wish to argue that the cluster of occupations comprising ancillary workers also enbraces a (more diluted) service ethic or ideology. The sociological literature of these occupations is very sparse; however, managerially oriented studies such as Dale's (1965) and the earlier Woodward (1950) have recently been supplemented by an extensive survey of ancillary workers' labour turnover in a group of London hospitals (Williams, Livy, Silverstone & Adams 1977). These indicate that porters, domestics and laundry workers are sharply conscious of their 'low status' as perceived by other groups of health service workers. As part of what may be a compensating occupational strategy they therefore seek to enhance the importance of their contribution to patient welfare and to value those aspects of their jobs which enable them to make this contribution.

... there is one aspect of hospital ancillary work that, as a number of reports show, is an important source of job satisfaction for many employees, namely, those tasks which lead to contact with patients. ... The rewarding nature of patient contact is perhaps one aspect of the broader concept of hospital ancillary work regarded as a 'worthwhile job', a job that enables the worker to feel that in some way he is being of service to the community.

Of course it will at once be argued that it makes no sense to treat porters and laundry workers, cooks and domestic staff as if they constituted an homogenous mass. It is probable that porters and domestics, having many opportunities for patient contact, will be more likely to advance status-enhancing claims about their role. However, in 1972, while observing negotiations about the implementation of Incentive Bonus Schemes for laundry staff in two separate Welsh Hospital Management Committee areas, I noted that both groups of staff advanced objections to the schemes on the grounds that a speed-up of production would result in a diminished quality of service to the patients.

Although there is an absence of data about NHS workers, a study of apartment-block janitors in the USA indicates that they stressed the 'responsible' nature of their jobs, and emphasised that the well-being and safety of large numbers of people were entrusted to their safekeeping. This, Gold (1964) concluded, was used as an occupational device to combat others' perceptions of their low-status job and generally to improve their image. In a later essay in the same volume Peter Berger (1964) talks of the 'pathetic confidence trick' of a hospital orderly employed in the removal of 'the repulsive debris of medical activity' styling himself a 'cuspidorologist'. Berger notes that this sleight-of-word is qualitatively no different from other strategies of occupational enhancement.

If it is once granted that both doctors and ancillary workers profess some form of ideology which has as a central component the ethic of service to the patient then the idea of a reflexive cost takes on a new dimension. Instead of representing merely the hardships involved in striking, or the degree of commitment to notions like 'solidarity', the health service worker is placed in a context of cognitive dissonance (Festinger 1962); that is, whatever tactics are mobilised publicly to support the official line that sanctions do not affect the well-being of the patient, there is a strong likelihood that the worker himself will perceive an incongruity between his service ideology and his behaviour. I do not contend that there is a deterministic cause-and-effect relationship between the ideology of service and the practitioner's actions. As Johnson (1972) puts it 'while the service ethic may be an important part of the ideology of many professional groups it is not clear that practitioners are necessarily so motivated'. Yet ideologies have a strongly moralistic content. 'An ideology', says MacIntyre (1971), 'is an account of the relationship between what is the case and how we ought to act.' One of the 'defining properties' of ideology is that 'it is not merely believed by a social group, but believed in such a way that it at least partially *defines for them their social existence*' (my emphasis). Thus, 'being a doctor' means, at least in part, being a person who defines himself as one who serves selflessly (even if in practice he might not). Taking industrial action, which can harm the patient, then, must place the professional's public definition of himself and his profession in question. It will be particularly difficult for doctors to support the continued use of such sanctions while maintaining their traditional professional concern for the well-being of their patients.

Analysis of any complicated industrial action is a forbidding task, while, as Richard Hyman points out, 'sensible generalisation is fraught with hazards'. It follows that hypothetical generalisation is foolhardy in the extreme. Nevertheless it seems impossible to leave this discussion without venturing a little further. David Mechanic points out some possibilities for professionals taking industrial action in a short study, 'Doctors in Revolt' (Mechanic 1974). He looked at the response of GPs to the BMA's call in 1965 for the submission of signed undated resignations from the NHS as a ploy in pay negotiations. Although Mechanic was specifically looking for factors involved in GPs' decisions to 'break the united medical front', he also noted that, since 'the threat of withdrawal from the health service conflicted with professional values a significant number of doctors probably felt some conflict when faced with a choice . . . there was some evidence that doctors with considerable "professional involvement" were less likely to submit resignations . . . we believe that men having these characteristics were more likely to hold strong professional values and therefore, experience greater conflict when faced with the resignation request'. It seems reasonable to suppose that this conflict will be enhanced if more overt sanctions are taken. Traditionally the threat of resignation from the NHS has been accompanied by tacit or explicit suggestions of *alternative* arrangements for health care systems. Strikes, of course, mean the absence of such an alternative.

Traditionally too, the medical profession in the UK has benefited greatly from its existing negotiating structure. Unlike the majority of other NHS staff, hospital doctors obtained, very early in the history of the NHS, dissolution of their Whitley Councils and the establishment of direct negotiations. Private discussions with the organ-grinder are more attractive, it seems, than public confrontation with the monkey. The evidence submitted by the BMA (and other professional associations representing doctors) to the successive independent Review bodies on Doctors' and Dentists' Remuneration (Pilkington, Halsbury, currently Woodroofe) indicates a wide spread of bargaining devices, including comparability arguments with other professionals within the UK, with doctors elsewhere in the world, especially America, the constant exodus of doctors to that and other promised lands, maintenance of differentials and so on. Public disputes of the kind we have been discussing radically narrow the range of deployable arguments; the issue becomes focused on confrontation. I have suggested that there are tactical dangers in taking this course.

One of the chief, perhaps unguessable, dangers relates to the tenuous 'contract' between professionals and the public they claim to serve. Alan Fox (1974) discusses the differing interpretations of 'trust' in occupational settings. He draws the common-sense distinction between 'trust' as the reposing of confidence in someone and the rather different implication of the kidnapper's reply to the question 'How do we know you'll do what you say?' 'You'll just have to trust me.' At the moment the trust generated between professional and patient is largely of the first kind, as we tend to accept professional valuations of their ethical and responsible attitudes to the public at their face value. Yet as Johnson, and Parry and Parry (among others) have pointed out, this claim to altruistic commitment is not proven. 'The fact that the men who write about the professions are usually professionals has meant that they have a tendency to project the justificatory ideology of professional men and their organisations' (Parry & Parry 1977:31).

Many have pointed out that claims to altruism are not easily tested. Industrial action might have the effect of disproving this claim; the claim to have the patient's interest at heart would also be severely questioned. Despite the fact that Illich and others have mounted a frontal attack on the mystique surrounding medical technology, one must agree with the Parrys that 'the prospect of de-professionalisation . . . seems to us to be an unlikely future for the medical profession in particular . . . '. Yet they ignore the equally frontal attack the profession seems itself to be mounting on that aspect of its mystique concerning the pre-eminence of the needs of the patient. They note that we may see 'doctors . . . relying increasingly in future upon union action rather than professionalism, however unpalatable this may be to those of the old guard in medicine who are ideologically antipathetic to unionism'. However, they fail to go on to consider precisely what factors are at stake, both for the always uneasy relationship between what doctors profess and what we see them do, and for the profession's valuation of its own codes of practice. It seems to me that industrial action of an overt kind places both these issues in an unusually bright and well-focused light. As Robinson (1973) notes, 'We assume that, as the health worker incorporates the values of his professional group and subjects himself to the evaluation of his colleagues, he is directed towards worthy goals and is insulated from improprieties.' By taking industrial action the health worker increases the risk of subjecting himself to public scrutiny of this assumption.

Acknowledgements

I would like to thank Peter Anthony, Paul Atkinson and Anne Murcott for their long-distance help. Without their assistance I can safely say this chapter would have been written but would not have had any references. I would also like to be able to claim that everything of merit is my own, and the mistakes are all other people's; I am afraid that the converse is probably true.

Finally, I would like to thank Nonna Jones for her patience and persistence in making sure that I almost met my deadlines.

12 THE SELF-HELP WAY TO HEALTH

Stuart Henry and David Robinson

> It matters not what you call them – self help, mutual aid,
> support systems – they are the fastest growing component of
> the human service industry. Nor is this surprising. Man is a
> social animal who throughout his history has banded together
> for problem solving and survival . . . Thus they are as old as
> man in one sense or a contemporary solution to complex
> problems in another. (Demone 1974:3)

We do not need Ivan Illich (1975) to persuade us that the complex
relationships between medical professionals, laymen and governments
are changing. Nor do we need reminding that money is tight and that
the range and scale of professional health and social services are being
curtailed, reorganised and generally rethought. Recent government
publications from several countries have emphasised the need for
personal responsibility in the prevention of illness and for greater
voluntary involvement in health care. In an interview with *The Times* in
February 1976, David Owen, then the British Minister of Health,
stressed the need for a fundamental shift toward a philosophy that:
'. . . health is not just something which is provided for . . . but that
each individual has a responsibility for his own well-being'. Not for
nothing was a Royal Commission on the National Health Services set up
in 1976. Not for nothing, either, has there been a rapid and substantial
increase in the number of self-help groups and organisations which,
taken together, now represent a significant feature of contemporary
life.

A good deal of attention has been given to self-help by both professionals and governments as well as by interested laymen and the
media. There are now self-help clearinghouses in both the United States
and the United Kingdom. There are self-help directories and there is
hardly any wide-circulation newspaper, magazine or professional journal
which has not carried an article on some aspect of self-help or on the
activities of some particular group. As well as the mainstream of self-
help groups there are other related developments which are often
referred to as part of the self-help movement. Among them are the
various volunteer schemes, the 'integrity' and other small groups
(Mowrer 1971), the growing number of self-treatment groups, self-

examination and self-care programmes which aim to lessen dependence
on the medical professions and, finally, there are the 'health by the
people' and other self-health developments in the third world which are,
at last, being written about (Newell 1975).

Self-help is clearly thought by many people to be a significant
feature of today's world. But it does not need to be spelled out that
people who share a certain problem might possibly have something to
offer each other. That 'something' might be emotional support,
material aid, friendship, technical expertise or a refuge from discrimination, hatred, stigma or quite simply 'the world out there'. So we must
not forget, in all the talk of a 'new' movement, that men have always
banded together to solve their problems or promote their activities, in
family networks, in clans and tribes, in guilds and professions, in trade
unions and friendly societies, in clubs and on street corners.

The best-known exposition of the Victorian philosophy of self-help
was written by Samuel Smiles. Published first in 1859, the preface to
the second edition of *Self-Help* contained Smiles' regret that some
people had misunderstood the book from its title and thought that he
was eulogising selfishness. He pointed out that, on the contrary, although its chief object was to stimulate self-reliance among the young
it was also the case that 'the duty of helping one's self in the highest
sense involves the helping of one's neighbours' (1866:iii). Almost a
hundred years later Professor Alan Moncrieff (1954) was moved to
inquire whether self-help was still alive, since benefits 'were to be
henceforth a right'. He felt that self-help was perhaps 'not dead but
sleeping'. In the next twenty years, however, self-help woke up, and
many people have written about its awakening.

Much of the literature on self-help has concentrated on the activities
of particular groups. Among the best-studied are alcoholics (Bean
1975), drug addicts (Yablonsky 1967), the overweight (Stunkard 1972),
little people (Weinberg 1968), widows (Silverman 1970), ex-mental
patients (Dean 1969), stutterers (Borkman 1974), parents without
partners (Harris 1966), parents of the handicapped (Katz 1961) and
deviants (Sagarin 1969). More recently, however, there have been a
number of attempts to draw together these accounts of particular
groups in order to find common aspects of their activity (Katz and
Bender 1976; Caplan and Killilea 1976). In this more general work,
writers have wrestled with the problems of how to define self-help
and how to classify self-help groups. Not surprisingly, given the wide
range of self-help enterprises with their differing origins, aims, philosophies, composition and political ideals, there are almost as many

definitions and classifications as there are groups (Killilea 1976).

We have not constructed any elaborate definitions or elegant typologies. Our aim has been to look at certain aspects of self-help activity which, on the basis of our study of self-help (Robinson and Henry 1977), appear to be particularly important. In this chapter we address three simple questions: Why self-help now? What is self-help? How does self-help work?

Why Self-Help Now?

Most answers to the question 'Why self-help now?' are couched in terms of a macro-cause-and-effect model which identifies self-help as a reaction to some inadequacy, need, problem or in some way changing situation. Some have argued that self-help is a response to the decline of existing institutions and the need to fill the gap. Mowrer (1971:45), for example, notes the decreasing importance of the established church and sees self-help groups as 'the emerging church of the 21st century'. Others see the decline in the extended family system and close-knit communities as bringing about a need for new ways of providing and sustaining emotional and social support (Weiss 1973; Wilson 1969).

Perhaps the most often heard 'failure of existing institutions' argument is that which takes the emergence of self-help to be a response to the disillusionment with the unfulfilled promise of the helping professions and the welfare state. Gussow and Tracy (1972:3), for example, assert that 'consumer-initiated services' arise when 'a hiatus exists between felt need and the existence of available services . . . adequate to meet such a need'. Others suggest, somewhat more sceptically, that the 'gaps' have arisen because of the inevitable fallibility of medical science and been aggravated by both the professionals' and the public's reluctance to acknowledge its failure. Zola (1975), for example, feels that many self-help groups grew up around those people who were abandoned by the medical services either because they represented its failings or because they had socially unacceptable problems.

In addition to arguments alleging the failure of traditional institutions there have been those which locate the growth of self-help in relation to changing philosophical, social and, in particular, psychiatric ideas. Glaser (1971), for example, suggests that self-help is a practical product of existential philosophy and learning theory. Zola (1975) notes its coincidence with a changing social conscience toward disablements following World War II, when previously unacceptable malaise became a national responsibility to which a social and economic commitment was made. Traunstein and Steinman (1973) have suggested that self-help is part of an alternative culture, reflected in a broader decentralisation, and debureaucratisation of public life. In the same vein, Vattano (1972) and Devall (1973) see self-help emerging as a power-to-the-people movement, itself a product of the cultural revolution of the 1960s and in a generally more tolerant political and social climate, while for Katz and Bender (1976) a mixture of these macro-social forces has combined to make self-help 'the most important social phenomenon in recent years'. They say that industrialisation, a money economy, the growth of vast structures of business, industry and government have led to: the depersonalisation and dehumanisation of institutions and social life, feelings of alienation, powerlessness, the loss of choices, and a loss of identity. Self-help is one of a number of social movements which, according to Katz and Bender, have arisen to counter this trend.

Groups' Accounts of their Origins

While global explanations may 'make sense', a greater understanding of 'Why self-help now?' may be gained from an examination of the emergence of particular groups. As part of our research, therefore, we analysed the voluminous literature produced by the self-help groups and organisations themselves, since a large proportion of them volunteer some account of how and why they formed.

It was clear from this that a whole range of people and agencies were in some way involved with the original setting up of the hundred and fifty different self-help groups which we looked at. There were the people who shared the problem, their intimates, various categories of professional and voluntary helpers, government departments, local authorities, community and voluntary agencies and the media. It was possible to abstract five major themes, issues or aspects of these groups' accounts which tended to recur. These were: (i) the identification of the shared problem, (ii) the failure of some agency, (iii) the recognition of the importance of meetings for those who share a common problem, (iv) innovations of some sort in handling the shared problem, and (v) the role of the media in bringing to light the extent of the shared problem, or some innovative attempt to solve it.

The stress given to any of these themes varied greatly from account to account. The most typical, however, as might be expected from the global explanations which were outlined earlier, was that which described people with a common problem meeting in a context of dissatisfaction with existing facilities and the idea to form a group being 'born'. As the Chairman of the Association for the Childless and Childfree said, this meeting proved rewarding because 'it helped people get off their chests the feeling of frustration and anger particularly about the medical side of fertility investigations, the problems of dealing with adoption and fostering agencies, and coping with the attitudes of relations and friends which was often critical or pitying'.

Almost half the accounts mentioned the media as playing a key role in some way. Depressives Associated, for example, started as a result of over 3,000 letters sent spontaneously in response to Nemone Lethbridge's television play *Baby Blues* which dealt with postnatal depression. Open Door was started in 1965 after a woman suffering from agoraphobia placed a small advertisement in a local newspaper and received a number of replies from other agoraphobics.

Some groups, such as the Ileostomy Association, the Society for Skin Camouflage, Possum Users Association and LIFT tie their origins to some professional innovation, while a small number of others say that they were set up to enable some professional to do what otherwise would have been impossible. Recovery Inc., for example, was started by Dr Abraham Low who felt he had to devise a more effective way of helping all the people who came to see him with their psychiatric problems. Recovery Inc. is interesting and unusual among the well-established self-help groups in its readiness to acknowledge the role of an outsider, and a professional at that, in its foundation (Antze 1976). But we must remember that we are dealing with histories; the purpose of which is to produce statements about the past which can be used in the present. And it may be more in line with beliefs about the nature and purpose of mutual self-help to drop references to the involvement of professionals and outsiders from accounts of time past. Which brings us to the second of our simple questions: 'What is self-help?'

What is Self-Help?

There has been a surprising lack of simple investigation into what self-help is, what self-help groups are and how they do what they do. Most of the literature produced by outsiders has done little more than say that self-help is either 'a good thing' or 'a bad thing'. Some, from a particular professional standpoint, have implied that self-help in some ways undermines their position. Koegler and Brill (1967:167), for example, emphasise the extremely charismatic approach of many self-help group leaders, bemoan the fact that the physician has lost much of *his* charisma in recent years, and conclude that in groups such as Alcoholics Anonymous and Synanon: 'there is a discounting of traditional authority, with an emphasis on the superior knowledge of the group and its leader'.

Fortunately, over the past few years, there have been a number of more serious attempts to analyse the nature of self-help and its place in the contemporary world. Rather than handing out lavish praise or voicing the worries of a profession under attack, writers such as Alfred Katz, and more recently Gerald Caplan and Maria Killilea (1976), have been gathering together the scattered literature in order to discover what self-help is taken to be and begin to describe what in practice self-help groups do. Killilea (1976) in her excellent review of the literature picks out certain *characteristics* of self-help groups which tend to be stressed. These are: *'Common experience of members'*; the belief that the care-giver has the same disability as the care-receiver, *'Mutual help and support'*; that the individual is a member of a group meeting regularly to provide mutual aid, *'The helper principle'*; that in a situation in which people help others with a common problem it may be the helper who benefits most from the exchange, *'Differential association'*; the reinforcement of self-concepts of normality hastening a person's separation from a previous deviant identity, *'Collective will-power and belief'*; the tendency to look to others in the group for validation, *'Importance of information'*; promotion of greater factual understanding of the problem and *'Constructive action toward shared goals'*; the notion that members learn and are changed by doing. That, however, is how 'outsiders' see self-help. What do members of self-help groups themselves think?

Members' Accounts

On the basis of the literature produced *by* the groups, they most typically see themselves as fellowships of people having the same problems and helping one another to overcome them through their own efforts and by sharing their experiences. Some self-help groups, in addition to 'problem sufferers', include among their membership professionals and 'interested non-professionals', such as friends and relatives. Most groups claim to be open to a wide variety of people: Families Need Fathers say they are 'open to men and women of any race, religion or creed who subscribe to the principles', while Recovery Inc. stress that their groups ' . . . are made up of adults from all walks of life — farmers, truck drivers, bankers, housewives, secretaries, artists, lawyers, doctors, businessmen, executives, clergymen and factory workers'.

But by far the most characteristic feature of the groups' self-images, is the stress put on the *common* problem, position, or circumstance;

colloquially expressed as 'being in the same boat'. This means, first of all, understanding the problems of others; that is, 'knowing what it's like'. It is said by numerous groups that only those experiencing the problem can *really* understand. 'Whatever the external help given by the State and statutory authorities', SHARE Community Ltd, a disablement group, the person will need understanding and encouragement, 'and these can best be given by those in a like case'. CARE, The Cancer Aftercare and Rehabilitation Society, say their organisation consists in the main of cancer patients, 'people who know what it is like to have cancer', and who they 'feel are best fitted to give moral assistance and help to patients and families before and after treatment'.

It is this *understanding* based on common experience, say the groups, which produces the necessary common bond of mutual interest and common desire to *do* something about the problem. And this 'doing something' is collectively helping oneself. As SHARE say about their organisation: 'It differs from practically all other organisations in the disablement field in that it aims not so much to do things for the disabled, as to help them to help themselves . . . '

In addition to these principles there is the repeated stress on the importance of 'example' in the sharing of experience and coping. The spirit of sharing is well summed up by the Association of Disabled Professionals who believe that it is a fundamental aim of their organisation that 'a battle fought successfully by one disabled person shall be a victory for all', and that 'those who follow in the successful path of existing members shall encounter fewer obstacles and far more encouragement and help on the journey'. As CARE explain, 'What better therapy than seeing someone who has had exactly what you have got, and who is . . . participating in all the normal activities of work and social life.' What better therapy indeed. But all these principles, while excellent statements of what self-help is, give little indication of how self-help groups actually do their self-help. Nor does it tell us why there is any need to do anything at all. In short, what is the problem?

Clearly, the range of problems, any one of which is shared in a particular self-help group, is immense. Many have been referred to already in this paper, and they may be physical, practical, mental, emotional, spiritual or social. For analytical purposes we consider them all under two heads: technical problems and social stigma. In any aspect of physical condition, mental well-being or social position or activity, there will be those who are technically abnormal, those with illnesses such as cancer, or who experience feelings of chronic depression, guilt or fear, or those whose interpersonal behaviour troubles them or others, or those with some social-situational problem such as being a single parent, or homeless, or a mental patient, or divorced.

Such technical problems, however, are not inherently problematic. While there may be practical difficulties, they may not be insurmountable. As an article in the magazine *Honey* (Brown 1976) explained, when discussing the Association for Research into Restricted Growth, 'the physical limitations of restricted growth are relatively easy to overcome — or at least learn to live with. Clothes can be made to measure and household appliances, and even cars, can be specially adapted to suit the little person's need: telephone kiosks, door handles and shaver points can, of course, present problems, but Mr. Pocock carries a neat briefcase which opens into two steps for just such eventualities.'

Clearly, what turns technical problems into major problems is that they cannot be handled by conventional problem-solving solutions. Also important is the way they are then interpreted by the people themselves, or by others.

Despite efforts to discount the discrediting attitudes of others, for example by saying that 'society doesn't understand', it is easy to see how, for many people, the combination of technical problems, failure of conventional problem-solving techniques and social stigma, assumes central and overwhelming importance. A member of Weight Watchers told us that to be slim 'was the only thing that mattered. It mattered to me passionately. It meant that when I was fat, wherever I went, I was conscious not of being a woman, nor . . . of being a something, or of being a friend, or of being a stranger. I was conscious only of being a fatty, and I felt ugly . . . Day and night for years it got me that bad.' Not surprisingly, the end result is to lose any sense of personal value. People describe themselves as feeling guilty and ashamed, feeling inadequate, having no identity, no confidence, no place in life, distressed, angry and finally, alone, since in the end there may be a gradual slide into secrecy, seclusion and isolation. How, then, does self-help work for people with these major problems?

How Does Self-Help Work?

At first glance, self-help groups appear to do so many different things for so many different purposes that any attempt at generalisation seems futile. On closer inspection, however, and with a degree of sensitive involvement, it becomes possible to identify a number of dominant themes and practices which play a significant role in the way self-help works.

Sharing

Sharing is the sharing of information and experience of the common problem, of coping with the common problem, and of successfully living again (cf. Wootton 1976). The mechanics of sharing range from formal group meetings where, as in AA, a crucial part is taken up with the telling of life stories, to no less important informal meetings between group members, telephone contact networks, correspondence and newsletters, or tape exchanges and radio contacts when the members are geographically dispersed or prevented by their shared problem from meeting face-to-face. In Touch, for example, a self-help group for the parents of mentally handicapped children, has a network of correspondence magazines consisting of letters from members; 'As each mother receives the magazine she reads all the other letters and replaces (her last one) with a new one commenting on the points raised.' These magazines circulate continuously so that each member gets up to a dozen letters every few weeks whilst writing only one.

The degree to which 'sharing' is explicitly recognised as a major feature of self-help activity varies from group to group. The crucial question about sharing is, how does it actually feature in the day-to-day working of self-help groups? Alcoholics Anonymous has recognised the importance of these questions. *Box 514* (1975), the AA newsletter, suggested that from time to time their members should re-examine what they meant by sharing – and what it is they are offering to share.

In self-help groups, sharing has two interrelated themes: we refer to these as deconstruction and reconstruction. *De*construction emphasises the group's attention to specific aspects of their common problems and how these are settled on, defused, dispersed, and generally coped with. *Re*construction emphasises those activities geared to the production of a new way of everyday life.

Self-help groups employ a variety of methods to relieve, manage or transform their members' problems. The first stage, though, is to enable and encourage people to identify and acknowledge that they 'are not alone with the problem'. It is easier for some people than for others. As Parents Anonymous, the self-help group for parents who abuse their children, say, 'the sooner you can share the nature of your problem and your concern for the problem, the sooner the other members will be able to relate to you in ways that will offer direct assistance'.

Paradoxically, perhaps, the 'deconstruction' of the problem initially involves concentrating on it. For a familiar part of self-help group work is to help people to settle, from among a whole complex of everyday problems of living, upon one clearly defined set of problems and agree that these are the central: admitting that one is 'an alcoholic', for example, or 'a child abuser'. Once this is done, a second stage of deconstruction can begin: the sharing of information about practical solutions to technical difficulties, such as providing physical aids, and information about official agencies and rights.

The third level of deconstruction, the most difficult, aims at destigmatisation: dispersing the perceived social discredibility of the members and their shared problems; a position nicely summarised by the National Association of the Childless and Childfree who believe that their members' common interest lies in 'trying to make it quite an unremarkable thing not to have children'.

One way of destigmatising the problem is by changing members' self-perception, a feat partly achieved by meeting others in the same situation, and, therefore, feeling less odd. It is quite common for groups to direct their destigmatising efforts towards changing those who are seen as the cause of teh stigma: 'the general public', or 'society', or just all those who 'do not understand'. In short, self-help groups aim to destigmatise the problem by changing both their members and outsiders. Thus the Campaign for Homosexual Equality 'provides a framework within which all women and men — whatever their sexual preference — can work together and . . . end all forms of discrimination against gay people . . . '.

As well as the relief of stigmatised problems, self-help groups can also provide recipes for an altered or *re*constructed life. At the same time they constitute a forum for putting those recipes into effect. The 'restructuring of life' is accomplished through doing projects together.

Project Work

It is difficult to generalise about projects, but basically they can be defined as co-operative activity, planned and organised by the members to achieve certain predetermined goals, and more or less explicit depending upon the particular group. Breakthrough Trust, for example, talk of 'integration projects with hearing people' such as going on outings, charity walks, holidays and holding jumble sales and dances. But no matter how elaborate or involving is a project, it is essential that it is important to the members. And clearly the most meaningful thing to the members is their problem, and so, naturally, most self-help project work is based on the core task of helping fellow members with their problems.

Indeed, Alcoholics Anonymous's whole programme can be seen as a collection of 'projects' designed to help fellow alcoholics. From merely telling his own drinking story at a group meeting, to twelfth-stepping and sponsoring newcomers, the AA member is actively helping fellow sufferers. In learning to tell his story appropriately, the newcomer is transforming devalued past experience into something useful (Bean 1975). It is a means of distancing the storyteller from the experience, and it is a personal example to use in the individual work of 'twelfth-stepping' and 'sponsorship'. As time goes on, the problem experience becomes only a part of a member's story. It is added to by reportable stages in AA group life, and by aspects of life outside the group which are contrasted with the 'problem' time before AA.

Time, and in particular the concentration on particular units or periods of time, is a recurrent theme in much self-help activity. Explicit distinctions are often made between time now and time past, between the member and his life now and in the past; while references to origins and 'the first time' are frequently made. Time is often formally structured in 'steps' and tightly maintained by group members and related to time targets which may be formally celebrated as in Gamblers Anonymous's 'Pin Night' or Weight Watchers' measuring of 'Goal Weight'. Time in the future is devalued while learning to live in the present, 'one day at a time', is stressed. Particular problems may be there 'for all time' and, since relapses can happen 'at any time', self-help commitment must be 'full-time'. To ensure self-help commitment is full-time, it is not enough for project work to be restricted to formal group meetings; it has to carry over into everyday life, and life outside the group.

Self-Help as a Way of Life

Most commentaries on self-help place too great an emphasis on group meetings. In successful self-help enterprises there is nearly always a certain amount of informal activity outside the formal meetings, which is not just incidental, but an essential part of the self-help process.

Some groups make it very explicit that their overall objective is to take the method of the group into the world outside, through the relationships which have been formed between group members. The intention is to transform the 'working' relationships in the group into friendships. Some groups, like AA and Parents Anonymous, increase the likelihood of friendship through their formal friendship or 'sponsorship' systems. Each new member is supposed to get a sponsor who acts in the way a close friend might.

One of the best ways of encouraging friendship is for people to engage in 'organised' *social*, rather than formal *group*, activities. Some branches of Gingerbread, the self-help group for one-parent families, arrange social activities every night, while others have them at least two or three times a week. Someone may hold a party. Someone else may organise a barbecue or a jumble sale or they might all go on holiday together. As their information officer told us, sharing a chalet with other people and their kids takes intimacy one step further; 'you're actually going to live with someone for a week, cooking together and everything else. A lot of friendships are really cemented during holidays.' The overall purpose of doing social projects, as Breakthrough Trust, for example, see more clearly than most, is to enable people to 'break through' the all embracing support of the self-help group to a new set of friendships and, thereby, to occupy a new place in the world, so that 'after a while', as the Chairman of The National Association for the Childless and Childfree explained, 'the groups become redundant because people have found groups of friends'.

The network of friendships fosters a feeling that help is always available. This is done by offering unsolicited help rather than waiting until a person asks for it. It would be peculiar for one's doctor to telephone 'out of the blue' and ask how you are, but in self-help helping that is exactly what happens. This ensures a feeling of the continuous availability, and even presence, of help, but also, by removing the onus of asking for help from the person with problems, it makes it quite an unremarkable thing both to have and be concerned about problems. It is here that self-help helping diverges most from conventional forms of help.

In self-help helping it is *not* a significant thing to ask for help. No appointments have to be made and there are no 'appropriate' times to 'phone or call. Help is given with pleasure when requested and offered spontaneously when not. There is no specialised knowledge possessed by by the helper that is denied to the helped. Those who are helpers are also friends. There is no distinction between treater and treated. All have problems. All are helpers. Because of this integration of helping and the helped, problem solvers and problem sufferers and friends, self-help helping merges into the everyday life of the member. Not only is self-help helping readily available, encouraged, and part of everyday life, but no restriction is placed on the *amount* of help which is given. As long as a person is in need of help he or she can have it. This is because the help is given out of personal concern and facilitated by a network of friendship.

Paradoxically, then, the significant part of self-help is that it makes both needing help, and helping, ordinary everyday things. From the very beginning of doing projects together, self-help becomes more than just something one does. Breakthrough Trust say that their integration projects bring about 'a dramatic change' in people. But it not just a *part* of people's lives that are changed. Accounts from group members suggest that the change is so dramatic that the person is changed completely: 'I had to change my whole outlook', said a Gamblers Anonymous member, 'I'm a different person.'

Self-help works for people whose problems are unsolvable by conventional means by transcending short-term solutions. In self-help groups, the problem is not separated off from everyday activities by buildings or chemicals. The treaters are not separated off by education, class or expertise. Nothing is hived-off, boxed away or cut out. In self-help helping the problem is integrated with life. Rather than living everyday life and having problems, self-help group members live their everyday life through their problems, which requires them to change their everyday lives.

Successful self-help groups, then, are much more than huddle-together sessions for people who feel discriminated against or overwhelmed by a common problem or by some aspect of late-twentieth-century life. The groups which offer most to their members are those which manage to combine mutual support for those who share a common problem with projects which enable people to build up a new set of relationships.

The women's self-health groups provide a good example of the way in which self-help can be an opportunity for growth rather than just a refuge from an unacceptable world. An important feature of self-health groups is for women to get to know, understand, monitor, respond to, control and appreciate the nature of the functioning of their own bodies. In the good groups this is only the beginning. The speculum is the instrument for opening up the passage not merely to one's cervix but to a new way of life. Linda Dove (1977), in a familiar declaration, succinctly makes the point when she says: 'Sometimes it seems that doctors and lovers have had more access to our bodies than we have. We must have power over our own bodies to control our lives.' That is the core of the self-help project method: to settle from among all the problems that one faces on a clear, understandable and manageable one, to 'find' that one can manage it and then to build a new life as a person who can control one's everyday problems and, thus, one's destiny. The project method, based on a shared appreciation of the need to structure time, is not just a matter of doing, it is a matter of *being*. It is a matter of being in the group, but it is also a matter of being outside the group. Self-help is a way of life. As the Founder of the Association for the Childless and Childfree put it: ' . . . just being together made us realize that being childless is . . . a chance for another kind of future based on finding the best in ourselves and offering it to others in whatever way appropriate.'

Self-Help and Health

Given the rapidly increasing interest in the whole field of self-help it is not surprising that the relationship between self-help and the established professions should have been discussed fairly extensively. First, there have been professionals themselves who, for the benefit of their colleagues, have attempted to identify the significance of self-help for everyday practice. Many have gone beyond emphasising the value of particular self-help enterprises to proposing that professionals should become directly involved. Vattano, for example, claims that there are certain functions which the professional is 'uniquely equipped to perform in self-help groups'. Jertson (1975), on the other hand, thinks such enthusiasm should be tempered, since it presents a number of problems which the facilitators ought to be aware of. He wonders whether professional involvement will ' . . . contribute to a loss of that one value uniquely cherished by the self-help group; the perceived ability to help itself'? He questions whether the groups will 'cease to be self-help if a professional organises and structures them'. He concludes that the role of facilitator is a most challenging task for the professional, but warns that it will demand 'a competent grasp of group theory and practice and, above all, a trusting capacity so that the professional, after organizing the group, is willing to let go'.

All this talk of whether or not professionals should or should not facilitate or otherwise get involved with self-help groups must not blind us to the fact that professionals as we have seen are, and always have been, intimately involved with even those self-help groups which are considered to be most independent and self-sufficient. Moreover, the members of many groups stress their close connections with, and the approval by, the medical and other professions.

At the beginning of this paper we drew attention to the fact that many commentators have seen the rapid growth of self-help groups as a new 'movement'. Some have waxed quite lyrical and seen the self-help phenomenon as a sign of the new Jerusalem. Vattano, for example, sees self-help groups as 'signs of en evolving more democratic society' while Dumont (1974) feels they represent 'a reification of the aspirations of the Founding Fathers, with their concern for individual rights, balance of power, and decentralization of power within pluralistic structures'. Such rhapsodical claims, however, do a grave injustice to the variety of self-help groups with their differing origins, activities, aims, philosophies and political stances. To suggest, as Vattano does, that self-help groups as a whole represent a form of counter-cultural protest with a 'power to the people' political stance is a gross and unhelpful simplification. As Katch (1975:6) argues, such a claim does not stand a moment's analysis; '. . . the aim of groups like AA . . . is exactly that of assisting their members to conform to the values of the dominant middle-class society.'

Whether or not we agree with Katz's assessment of AA, he is absolutely right to call for 'sharper' analysis, which attempts 'to understand the phenomena with which we are dealing in the many-sidedness'. For it is only by looking at what self-help groups actually do that we can hope to get away from catchy but unilluminating slogans and begin to appreciate what, at ground level, self-help *is* for particular people with particular problems. For self-help groups are of interest today, not merely because governments are short of money — which, of course, they are — or because the groups are symbols of anti-professionalism — which, of course, they may be — but because some of them actually work. The sooner professionals, laymen and governments rediscover the simple fact that those who share a certain illness, disability, problem or position in the world have something to offer each other, whether that 'something' is emotional support, technical expertise, a refuge from the discrimination or stigma, or a new way of life, the sooner we will experience the real meaning of health.

BIBLIOGRAPHY

Abel-Smith, B. (1964). *The Hospitals 1800-1948*. London: Heinemann

Abrams, M. (1959). *The Teenage Consumer*. London: Press Exchange

Abrams, P. (1977). Community Care: Some Research Problems and Priorities. *Policy and Politics* 6: 125-51

Adelstein, A.M. (1952). Accident Proneness: A Criticism of the Concept Based on an Analysis of Shunters' Accidents. *Journal of the Royal Statistical Society* 115: 111

Andrews, C.J. (1975). *The First Cornish Hospital*. No publishing data given: Printed Penzance

Anthony, P.D. and Crichton, A. (1969). *Industrial Relations and the Personnel Specialist*. London: Batsford

Antze, P. (1976). The Role of Ideologies in Peer Psychotherapy Organisations: some theoretical considerations and three case studies. *Journal of Applied Behavioural Science* 12: 323-46

Atkinson, P. (1977). The Reproduction of Medical Knowledge. In R. Dingwall *et al.* (eds.) *Health Care and Health Knowledge*. London: Croom Helm

Austin, R. (1976). *Occupation and Profession in the Organisation of Nursing Work*. Unpublished PhD Thesis. University of Wales

—— (1978). The Nurse Practitioner in Health Care. *International Nursing Review* 25: 82-8

Barber, B. (1963). Some Problems in the Sociology of Professions. *Daedalus* 92: 669-88

Barker, D.L. and Allen, S. (eds.) (1976). *Dependence and Exploitation in Work and Marriage*. Harlow: Longmans

Bayley, M. (1973). *Mental Handicap and Community Care*. London: Routledge and Kegan Paul

Beales, T.G. *et al.* (1976). *The Microcosm: Health Centres in Practice*. Bradford: Organisational Analysis Research Unit, Management Centre, University of Bradford

Bean, M. (1975). *Alcoholics Anonymous*. New York: Psychiatric Annals Reprint

Bell, J. and Redwood, T. (1880). *Historical Sketch of the Progress of Pharmacy in Great Britain*. London: Pharmaceutical Society

Berger, P.L. (1964). *The Human Shape of Work*. New York: Macmillan

—— (1964). Some General Observations on the Problem of Work. In

P.L. Berger (ed.) *The Human Shape of Work.* New York: Macmillan

Bernstein, B. (1970). Education Cannot Compensate for Society. *New Society* 26 February: 344-7

—— (1975). *Class, Codes and Control Vol. 3.* London: Routledge and Kegan Paul

Beveridge Report (1942). *Social Insurance and Allied Services.* Report by Sir William Beveridge. Cmd. 6404

Beynon, H. (1973). *Working for Ford.* Harmondsworth: Penguin

Blaxter, M. (1976). Social Class and Health Inequalities. In C.O. Carter and J. Peel (eds) *Equalities and Inequalities in Health.* London: Academic Press

Bluck, M.E. (1975). *Public and Professional Opinion on Preventive Medicine.* Cardiff: Tenovus Cancer Information Centre

Borkman, T. (1974). A Cross-National Comparison of Stutterers' Self-help Organisations. *New Zealand Speech Therapy Journal* 29: 6-16

Bott, E. (1971). *Family and Social Network.* London: Tavistock

Bouer, H. (1971). To Diagnose or Not to Diagnose: A Naive Inquiry. *International Journal of Group Psychotherapy* 21: 470-5

British Medical Association (BMA) (1946). *A Charter for Health.* London: Allen and Unwin

—— (1961). *The Future of the Occupational Health Services:* Report of a Working Party. London

Brockington, F. (1954). *The Health of the Community.* London: Churchill

Brown, A. (1976). Big Problems for Little People. *Honey* February: 10-11

Brown, C.W. and Ghiselli, E.E. (1948). Accident Proneness Among Streetcar Motormen and Motor Coach Operators. *Journal of Applied Psychology* 32: 20

Brunsdon, C. (1978). It is Well Known that Women are Inclined to be Rather Personal. In Womens' Studies Group, *Women Take Issue.* London: Hutchinson

Bucher, R. and Stelling, J.L. (1977). *Becoming Professional.* Beverly Hills: Sage Publications

Calder, A. (1971). *The People's War.* London: Panther

Caplan, G. and Killilea, M. (eds.) (1976). *Support Systems and Mutual Help: Multidisciplinary Explorations.* New York: Grune and Stratton Inc.

Carpenter, M. and Fairclough, A. (1977). Paid and Unpaid Labour. Unpublished paper presented to Medical Sociology Workshop,

University of Warwick

Carr-Saunders, A.M. and Wilson, P.A. (1933). *The Professions.* Oxford: Oxford University Press

Carsen, C.O. and Peel, J. (1976). *Equalities and Inequalities in Health.* London: Academic Press

Cartwright, A. (1970). *Parents and Family Planning Services.* London: Routledge and Kegan Paul

Castle, B. (1975). *NHS Revisited.* Pamphlet based on Nye Bevan Memorial Lecture, Oxford. Fabian Tract 440. London: Fabian Society

Central Health Services Council (1969). *The Functions of the District General Hospital.* London: HMSO. (Bonham-Carter Report)

Committee of Enquiry into Health, Safety and Welfare in Non-Industrial Employment (1949). *Report.* Cmnd. 7664. London: HMSO. (Gower Report)

Committee of Enquiry on Industrial Health Services (1951). *Report.* Cmnd. 8170. London: HMSO. (Dale Report)

Committee on Local Authority and Allied Personal Social Services (1968). *Report.* Cmnd. 3703. London: HMSO. (Seebohm Report)

Cooper, M.H. and Culyer, A.J. (1972). Equality in the NHS: Intentions, Performance and Problems in Evaluation. In M. Hauser (ed.) *The Economics of Medical Care.* London: Allen and Unwin

Cooper, M.H. (1975). *Rationing Health Care.* London: Croom Helm

Coote, A. and Gill, T. (1977). *Women's Rights: a Practical Guide.* Harmondsworth: Penguin

Council for the Education and Training of Health Visitors (CETHV) (1977). *An Investigation into the Principles of Health Visiting*

Cox, C. and Mead, A. (eds.) (1975). *A Sociology of Medical Practice.* London: Collier-Macmillan

Crellin, J.K. (1967). The Growth of Professionalism in 19th Century British Pharmacy. *Medical History* 11

Crossman, R. (1972). *A Politician's View of Health Service Planning.* Glasgow: University of Glasgow

Curwen, M. and Brookes, B. (1969). Health Centres: Facts and Figures. *The Lancet* 2: 945-8

Dale, A.J. (1965). Job Satisfaction and Organisation Among Hospital Domestic Workers. *British Journal of Industrial Relations* 3 (2)

Davidoff, L., L'Esperance, J. and Newby, H. (1976). Landscape with Figures: Home and Community in English Society. In J. Mitchell and A. Oakley (eds.) *The Rights and Wrongs of Women.* Harmondsworth: Penguin

Dean, S.R. (1969). Recovery Inc., Giving Psychiatry an Assist. *Medical Economics* 2 September

Demone, H.W. Jnr. (1974). *Introduction to Directory of Mutual Help Organisations in Massachusetts* (4th ed.). Massachusetts: Blue Cross and Blue Shield

Department of Employment (1972). *Safety and Health at Work.* London: HMSO. Cmnd. 5034. (Robens Report)

Department of the Environment (DoE) (1975). *National Travel Survey 1972/73, Part 1.* London: HMSO

Department of Health and Social Security (DHSS) (1970). *Report on the Hospital Pharmaceutical Service.* London: HMSO (Noel Hall Report)

——(DHSS) (1971). *Better Services for the Mentally Handicapped.* Cmnd. 4683. London: HMSO

——(1975). *Better Services for the Mentally Ill.* Cmnd. 6233. London: HMSO

——(1976a). *Prevention and Health: Everybody's Business. A Reassessment of Public and Personal Health.* London: HMSO

——(1976b). *Health and Personal Social Services Statistics.* London: HMSO

——(1976c). *Priorities for Health and Personal Social Services in England: A Consultative Document.* London: HMSO

——(1976d). *Annual Report of the Department of Health and Social Security 1975.* London: HMSO

——(1977a). *Smoking and Professional People.* London: HMSO

——(1977b). Proceedings of the Symposium 'Prevention and Health' July 1976. London

——(1977c). *The Way Forward.* London: HMSO

——(1977d). *Prevention and Health.* Cmnd. 7047. London: HMSO

Devall, B. (1973). Gay Liberation: An Overview. *Journal of Voluntary Action Research* 2: 24-35

Dicey, A.C. (1905). *Lectures on the Relation between Law and Public Opinion in England During the Nineteenth Century.* London: Macmillan

Dingwall, R. (1974). *The Social Organisation of Health Visitor Training.* Unpublished PhD Thesis. University of Aberdeen

——(1976). *Aspects of Illness.* London: Martin Robertson

——(1977a). Collectivism, Regionalism and Feminism: Health Visiting and British Social Policy 1850-1975. *Journal of Social Policy* 6: 291-315

——(1977b). *The Social Organisation of Health Visitor Training.*

London: Croom Helm

Dove, L. (1977). Self-Help Centres in Los Angeles. *Spare Rib* 55: 26-7

Draper, P. (1976). The Organisation of Health Care: A Critical View of the 1974 Reorganisation of the NHS. In D. Tuckett (ed.) *An Introduction to Medical Sociology.* London: Tavistock

—— et al. (1976). *Health, Money and the NHS.* London: Unit for the Study of Health Policy, Guy's Hospital, London

Dubos, R. (1959). *The Mirage of Health.* New York: Harper

Dumont, M.P. (1974). Self-Help Treatment Programs. *American Journal of Psychiatry* 131: 631-5

Eckstein, H. (1958). *The English Health Service.* Cambridge, Mass.: Harvard University Press

Elston, M.A. (1977). Medical Autonomy: Challenge and Response. In K. Barnard and K. Lee (eds.) *Conflicts in the National Health Service.* London: Croom Helm

Ennals, D. (1977). Better Value for Money in the NHS. *Rehabilitation* January-March 100: 41-9

Etheridge, J.I.B. (1976). Health Centre Circumstances, Past and Present. In J.G. Beales *et al. The Microcosm: Health Centres in Practice.* Organisational Analysis Research Unit, Management Centre, University of Bradford

Ferguson, M. (1978). A Canadian Way. *Nursing Times* 13 July

Festinger, L. (1962). *When Prophecy Fails.* New York: Harper Row

Foreman, A. (1977). *Femininity as Alienation: Women and the Family in Marxism and Psychoanalysis.* London: Pluto

Forsyth, G. (1973). *Doctors and State Medicine.* London: Pitman Medical. 2nd ed.

Foucault, M. (1973). *The Birth of the Clinic.* London: Tavistock

Fox, A. (1974). *Beyond Contract: Work, Power and Trust Relations.* London: Faber

Freidson, E. (1970). *Profession of Medicine.* New York: Dodd Mead

Gardiner, J. (1976). Political Economy of Domestic Labour in Capitalist Society. In D.L. Barker and S. Allen (eds.) *Dependence and Exploitation in Work and Marriage.* Harlow: Longmans

General Medical Council (1977). *A Survey of Basic Medical Training.* Oxford: Nuffield Provincial Hospitals Trust

Gilbert, B.B. (1966). *The Evolution of National Insurance in Great Britain: The Origins of the Welfare State.* London: Michael Joseph

Glaser, F. (1971). Gandenzia Incorporated: Historical and Theoretical Background of a Self-Help Addiction Treatment Program. *International Journal of Addictions* 6: 615-26

Glover, J. (1977). *Causing Death and Saving Lives.* Harmondsworth: Penguin

Gold, R. (1964). In the Basement – the Apartment Building Janitor. In P.L. Berger (ed.) *The Human Shape of Work.* New York: Macmillan

Goldthorpe, J.H. and Lockwood, D., *et al.* (1969). *The Affluent Worker in The Class Structure.* Cambridge University Press

Goodman, P. (1961). *Growing up Absurd.* London: Victor Gollancz

Gorshenon, C. (1970). Trends in Health Care. *Maternal and Child Health Information* 4

Gove, W.R. (1972). The Relationship Between Sex Roles, Marital Roles and Mental Illness. *Social Forces* 51: 34-44

―― and Tudor, J.F. (1973). Adult Sex Roles and Mental Illness. *American Journal of Sociology* 78, 4: 812-35

Gove, W.R. (1973). Sex, Marital Status and Mortality. *American Journal of Sociology* 79, 1:45-67

Gregory, D. and McCarty, J. (1975). *The Shop Steward's Guide to Health and Safety at Work.* Nottingham: Spokesman Books

Guillebaud (1956). See Ministry of Health (1956)

Gussow, Z. and Tracy, G. (1972). *A Prospectus of Voluntary Self-Help Health Organisations: A Study in Human Support Systems.* New Orleans: Louisiana State University

Hall, S. and Jefferson, T. (eds.) (1975). *Resistance Through Rituals.* London: Hutchinson

Halmos, P. (1970). *The Personal Service Society.* London: Constable

Harris, A. and Clausen, R. (1966). *Labour Mobility in Britain 1953-63.* An enquiry undertaken for the Ministry of Labour and National Service in 1963. London: HMSO

Harris, E.T. (1966). Parents without Partners Inc.: A Resource for Clients. *Social Work* 11: 92-8

Hart, N. (1978). *Health and Inequality.* University of Essex. Mimeo.

Hauser, M. (ed.) (1972). *The Economics of Medical Care.* London: Allen and Unwin

Health and Safety Commission (1977). *Occupational Health Services: The Way Ahead.* London: HMSO

Heller, T. (1978). *Restructuring the Health Service.* London: Croom Helm

Hodgkinson, R.G. (1967). The Origins of the NHS: The Medical Services of the New Poor Law 1834-71. Wellcome Historical Medical Library. *Historical Monograph Series* 11

Hoggart, R. (1958). *The Uses of Literacy.* Harmondsworth: Penguin

Hollingshead, A.B. and Redlich, F.C. (1958). *Social Class and Mental Illness.* New York: Wiley

Hospital Group of the Pharmaceutical Society of Great Britain (1977). *Forum on Clinical Pharmacy.* London

Hulka, B.S., Cassel, J.C., Kupper, L.L. and Burdette, J.A. (1976). Communication, Compliance, and Concordance between Physicians and Patients with Prescribed Medications. *American Journal of Public Health* 66: 847-53

Hyman, R. (1972). *Strikes.* Glasgow: Fontana

Iliffe, S. and Gordon, H. (1977). *Pickets in White.* London: Medical Practitioners Union

Illich, I. (1975). *Medical Nemesis: The Expropriation of Health.* London: Calder and Boyars

—— (1976). *Limits to Medicine.* London: Marion Boyars

Illsley, R. (1976). Everybody's Business? Concepts of Health and Illness. SSRC Health and Health Policy Panel

Isaacs, S. (1941). *The Cambridge Evacuation Survey.* London: Methuen

Jertson, J. (1975). Self-Help Groups. *Social Work* 20: 144-5

Jewkes, J. and S. (1963). *Value for Money in Medicine.* Oxford: Basil Blackwell.

Johnson, T.J. (1972). *Professions and Power.* London: Macmillan

Jordan, B. (1976). *Freedom and the Welfare State.* London: Routledge and Kegan Paul

Katz, A. (1961). *Parents of the Handicapped.* Springfield, Illinois: Charles C. Thomas

—— (1975). Some Thoughts on Self-Help Groups and the Professional Community. Paper Presented to National Conference on Social Welfare, San Francisco, May

Katz, A.H. and Bender, E.I. (eds.) (1976). *The Strength in Us: Self-Help Groups in the Modern World.* New York: Franklin Watts

Killilea, M. (1976). Mutual Help Organisations: Interpretations in the Literature. In Caplan, G. and Killilea, M. (eds.) *Support Systems and Mutual Help: Multidisciplinary Explorations.* New York: Grune & Stratton Inc. 37-93

Klein, R. (1973). *Complaints Against Doctors: A Study in Professional Accountability.* London: Charles Knight

—— (ed.) (1975). *Social Policy and Public Expenditure 1975: Inflation and Priorities.* Centre for Studies in Social Policy

—— (1977). Policy Options for Medical Manpower. *British Medical Journal* 9 July: 136-7

—— *et al.* (1974). *Social Policy and Public Expenditure, 1974.* Centre for Studies in Social Policy

Koegler, R.R. and Brill, N.Q. (1967). *Treatment of Psychiatric Out-Patients.* New York: Appleton-Century-Crofts

Komarovsky, M. (1967). *Blue Collar Marriage.* New York: Vintage Books

Lane, T. (1975). *The Union Makes Us Strong.* London: Arrow

Lapping, A. (1970). Community Careless. *New Society* 9 April

Leninger, M. (1975). An Open Health Care System Model. In B.W. Spradley (ed.) *Contemporary Community Nursing.* Boston: Little Brown

Lipsey, R.G. (1966). *An Introduction to Positive Economics.* (2nd ed.) London: Weidenfeld and Nicholson

McFarlane, J. (1976). The Role of Research and the Development of Nursing Theory. Paper delivered to Royal College of Nursing (RCN) Research Society

McGlothlin, W.J. (1964). *The Professional Schools.* New York. The Center for Applied Research in Education

MacIntyre, A. (1971). The End of Ideology and the End of the End of Ideology. In A. MacIntyre (1971) *Against the Self-Images of the Age.* London: Duckworth

McKeown, T. (1971). A Historical Appraisal of the Medical Task. In G. McLachlan and T. McKeown (eds.) (1971) *Medical History and Medical Care.* Nuffield Provincial Hospital Trust. Oxford University Press

——— (1976). *The Role of Medicine: Dream, Mirage or Nemesis?* London: Nuffield Pronvincial Hospital Trust

McLachlan, G. and McKeown, T. (eds.) (1971). *Medical History and Medical Care.* Nuffield Provincial Hospital Trust Oxford University Press

Mayer, J. and Timms, N. (1969). Clash in Perspective Between Worker and Client. *Social Casework* January: 32-40

Mayers, M.G. (1973). *A Systematic Approach to the Nursing Care Plan.* New York: Appleton

Maynard, A. and Walker, A. (1977). Too Many Doctors? *Lloyds Bank Review* July: 24-36

Meacher, M. (1972). *Taken for a Ride.* Harlow: Longmans

Mechanic, D. (1974). Doctors in Revolt: The Crisis in the English NHS. In. D. Mechanic, *Politics, Medicine and Social Science.* New York: Wiley

——— (1974). *Politics, Medicine, and Social Science.* New York: Wiley

Millerson, G. (1964). *The Qualifying Associations.* London: Routledge and Kegan Paul

Ministry of Health (1944). *A National Health Service. The White Paper Proposals in Brief.* London: HMSO

—— (1956). *Report of the Committee of Enquiry into the Cost of the NHS.* London: HMSO. (Guillebaud Report)

—— (1962). *A Hospital Plan for England and Wales.* London: HMSO

—— (1963). *Health and Welfare: The Development of Community Care.* London: HMSO

—— (1966). *Report of the Committee on Senior Nursing Staff Structure.* London: HMSO. (Salmon Report)

—— (1967). *On the State of the Public Health.* London: HMSO

Ministry of Labour and National Service (1956). Staffing and Organisation of the Factory Inspectorate. London: HMSO

Mitchell, J. and Oakley, A. (eds.) (1976). *The Rights and Wrongs of Women.* Harmondsworth: Penguin

Moncrieff, A. (1954). The Meaning of Self-Help in Social Welfare. In *Self-Help and Social Welfare. Proceedings of the Seventh International Conference of Social Welfare.* Bombay: SE Asia Regional Office of the International Conference of Social Work

Moroney, R. (1976). *The Family and the State.* Harlow: Longman

Morris, J.N. (n.d.). *Health.* No. 6, Books for Discussion Groups. Published for the Association for Education in Citizenship by the English University Press

Mowrer, O.H. (1971). Peer Groups and Medication: The Best 'Therapy' for Laymen and Professionals Alike. *Psychotherapy: Theory, Research and Practice* 8: 44-54

Nathanson, C.A. (1975). Illness and the Feminine Role. A Theoretical Review. *Social Science and Medicine* 9: 57-62

Navarro, V. (1976). *Medicine Under Capitalism.* London: Croom Helm

Newell, J.N. (ed.) (1975). *Health by the People.* Geneva: World Health Organisation

Newson, J. and E. (1970). Four Years Old in an Urban Community. Harmondsworth: Penguin Books

Oakley, A. (1974a). *The Sociology of Housework.* London: Martin Robertson

—— (1974b). *Housewife.* Harmondsworth: Penguin Books

—— (1976). The Family, Marriage and Its Relationship to Illness. In David Tuckett (ed.) *An Introduction to Medical Sociology.* Tavistock

Office of Population, Census and Surveys (OPCS) (1975). *General Household Survey 1973.* London: HMSO

—— (1974). *Morbidity Statistics from General Practice.* 2nd National
Study 1970-71. Studies on Medical and Population Subjects No. 26.
London: HMSO

—— (1975). *Mortality Statistics; Cause.* Reports for Years 1970-75.
London: HMSO

Owen, D. (ed.) (1968). *A Unified Health Service.* Oxford: Pergamon
Press

—— (1976). *In Sickness and in Health.* London: Quartet

Parry, N. and Parry, J. (1977). *The Rise of the Medical Profession.*
London: Croom Helm

Pavitt, L. (1963). *The Health of the Nation.* London: Fabian Society

Pelz, D.C., McDole, T.L., Schuman, S.H. (1975). Drinking-Driving
Behaviour of Young Men in Relation to Accidents. *Journal of
Studies on Alcohol* July 36(7): 956-72

Pharmaceutical Society of Great Britain (1977). Evidence to the Royal
Commission on the National Health Service. *Pharmaceutical Journal*
25 September

Porter, A. (1970). Depressive Illnes in a General Practice: A Demographic Study and a Controlled Trial of Imipramine. *British Medical
Journal* 1: 773-8

Poston, J.W. (n.d.). Department of Pharmacy, UWIST, Cardiff.
Personal Communication

Powell, E. (1966). *Medicine and Politics.* London: Pitman

Powles, J. (1972). On the Limitations of Modern Medicine. *Science,
Medicine and Man* 1

Radical Statistics Health Group (1976). *Whose Priorities?* London:
Radical Statistics

Rainwater, L. (1960). *And the Poor Get Children.* Chicago: Quadrangle

Roberts, F. (1952). *The Cost of Health.* London: Turnstile Press

Robinson, D. (1973). *Patients, Practitioners and Medical Care.* London:
Heinemann

—— and Henry, S. (1977). *Self-Help and Health.* London: Martin
Robertson

Robson, J. (1972). *Take a Pill . . . The Drug Industry – Private or
Public.* London: Marxists in Medicine

Ross, J.S. (1952). *The National Health Service in Great Britain.*
London: Oxford University Press

Royal Commission on Medical Education (1968). *Report.* Cmnd. 3569.
London: HMSO.(Todd Report)

Roy-Chowdhury, S. (1977). Medical Assistants: Britain's Cinderella
Consultants. *Sunday Times* 3 July

Sagarin, E. (1969). *Odd Man In: Societies of Deviants in America.* Chicago: Quadrangle Books

Shetland, M.L. (1975). An Approach to Role Expansion. In B.W. Spradley (ed.) *Contemporary Community Nursing.* Boston: Little Brown

Silverman, P.R. (1970). The Widow as Caregiver in a Program of Preventive Intervention with Other Widows. *Mental Hygiene* 54:540-7

Smiles, S. (1866). *Self-Help: With Illustrations of Character, Conduct and Perseverance.* London: Murray (2nd ed.)

Smith, M.C. and Knapp, D.A. (1972). *Pharmacy, Drugs and Medical Care.* Baltimore: Williams and Wilkins

Sorsby, A. (1942). *Medicine and Mankind.* London: Scientific Book Club

Spradley, B.W. (ed.) (1975). *Contemporary Community Nursing.* Boston: Little Brown

Stevens, R. (1966). *Medical Practice in Modern England.* New Haven: Yale University Press

Strange, M.H. (1962). *Modern English Structures.* London: Edward Arnold

Strong, P.M. (1978). Professional Medicine, Professional Sociology and Medical Imperialism. MRC Medical Sociology Unit, Aberdeen. Mimeo

—— and Horobin, G.W. (1977). Politeness is All – The Forms, Causes and Consequences of Medical Gentility. Institute of Medical Sociology, Aberdeen. Mimeo

Stunkard, A.J. (1972). The Success of TOPS, a Self-Help Group. *Postgraduate Medicine* May, 144-7

Tax, S. (1975). *Topias and Utopias in Health.* Denver: Morton

The Todd Report (1968). Report of the Royal Commission on Medical Education. April. Cmnd. 3569. London: HMSO

Tisdall, C. (1976). Artists' Co-op. *The Guardian* 12 March

Titmuss, R.M. (1958). *Essays on the Welfare State.* London: Allen and Unwin

Tones, B.K. (1977). *Effectiveness and Efficiency in Health Education. A Review of Theory and Practice.* Occasional Paper. Scottish Health Education Unit

Townsend, P. (1974). Inequality and the Health Service. *The Lancet* 15 June

Trades Union Congress (1945). Annual Congress Report

—— (1969). Annual Congress Report

Traunstein, D.M. and Steinman, R. (1973). Voluntary Self-Help Organisation: an Exploratory Study. *Journal of Voluntary Action Research* 2: 230-9

Tuckett, D. (ed.) (1976). *An Introduction to Medical Sociology.* London: Tavistock

Tudor Hart, J. (1971). The Inverse Care Law. *The Lancet* 27 February

UICC (1977). *Lung Cancer Prevention, Guidelines for Smoking Control.* Geneva: Centre Internationale de Cancer

United States Department of Health, Education and Welfare (HEW) (1970). *Selected Symptoms of Psychological Stress.* National Council for Health Statistics

Vance, P.H. (1973). The Effect of a Pharmaceutical Drug Surveillance Program in an Acute Ward. *Canadian Journal of Hospital Pharmacy* 26, March/April

Van Zelst, R.H. (1954). Effect of Age and Experience Upon Accident Rate. *Journal of Applied Psychology* 38: 313

Vattano, A. (1972). Power to the People: Self-Help Groups. *Social Work* 17: 7-15

Waddington, I. (1973). The Role of the Hospital in the Development of Modern Medicine: A Sociological Analysis. *Sociology* 7: 211-24

—— (1977). General Practitioners and Consultants in Early Nineteenth-Century England. In J. Woodward and D. Richards (eds.) *Health Care and Popular Medicine in Nineteenth Century England.* London: Croom Helm

Wakefield, J. and Sansom, C.D. (1966). Profile of a Population of Women Who Have Undergone a Cervical Smear Examination. *The Medical Officer* 116: 145-6

Waldron, I. (1976). Why Do Women Live Longer Than Men? *Social Science and Medicine* 10: 349-62

Walton, R.E. and McKersie, R.B. (1965). *A Behavioural Theory of Labour Negotiations.* New York: McGraw Hill

Webb, S. and Webb, B. (1910). *The State and The Doctor.* London: Longmans, Green and Co.

Weinberg, M.S. (1968). The Problems of Midgets and Dwarfs and Organisational Remedies. *Journal of Health and Social Behaviour* 9: 65-72

Weiss, R.S. (1973). Parents Without Partners as a Supplementary Community. In R.S. Weiss (ed.) *Loneliness: the Experience of Emotion and Social Isolation.* Cambridge, Mass.: MIT Press

Weiss, R.S. (1973). *Loneliness: the Experience of Emotional and Social Isolation.* Cambridge, Mass.: MIT Press

Wertheimer, A.I. and Smith, M.C. (1974). *Pharmacy Practice.* Baltimore:

University Park Press

Willcocks, A.J. (1967). *The Creation of the NHS: A Study of Pressure Groups and a Major Policy Decision.* London: Routledge and Kegan Paul

Wilson, A. (1969). Self-Help Groups: Rehabilitation or Recreation. *American Journal of Correction.* November-December: 12-13

Wilson, E. (1977). *Women and the Welfare State.* London: Tavistock

Wilson, M. (1975). *Health is for People.* London: Darton, Longman and Todd

Women's Studies Groups (1978). *Women Take Issue.* Centre for Contemporary Cultural Studies, University of Birmingham. Hutchinson

Woodward, J. (1950). *Employment Relations in a Group of Hospitals.* London: Institute of Hospital Administrators

—— (1974). *To Do the Sick No Harm.* London: Routledge and Kegan Paul

—— and Richards, D. (eds.) (1977). *Health Care and Popular Medicine in Nineteenth Century England.* London: Croom Helm

Wootton, A. (1977). Sharing: Some Notes on the Organisation of Talk in a Therapeutic Community. *Sociology* 11: 333-50

Yablonsky, L. (1967). *Synanon: The Tunnel Back.* Baltimore: Penguin Books

Young, M. and Willmott, P. (1973). *The Symmetrical Family.* London: Routledge and Kegan Paul

Zaretsky, E. (1976). *Capitalism, the Family and Personal Life.* London: Pluto

Zola, I. (1975). Helping One Another: a Brief History of Mutual Aid Groups. Brandeis University. Mimeo.

CONTRIBUTORS

Paul Atkinson Lecturer in Sociology, University College Cardiff. Present interests include health, fitness and schooling and ethnographic research methods.

Rita Austin Assistant Registrar in the Council for National Academic Awards. She has completed doctoral work on the social context of nursing work and has published in nursing journals. Her present research interests are concerned with developing theories of practice.

Max Blythe Education Adviser and Co-ordinator for Health Education in Oxfordshire. A biologist, he taught in schools and in higher education, and is currently Awarder in A Level Biology for the Oxford and Cambridge Examinations Board. He has published scientific papers on biological subjects and is currently editing a series of biology texts for the Web of Life series of publications by Longmans.

Celia Davies Senior Research Fellow in Sociology at Warwick University. She is currently working on the history of nursing in Britain and America. Her interests include the sociology of professions, and the history of health care institutions and organisations.

Robert Dingwall At the SSRC Centre for Socio-Legal Studies, Oxford, working on a study of child protection. His previous work, with the Institute of Medical Sociology in Aberdeen, was concerned with health visiting and with physically disabled teenagers. He has published books on health visiting and concepts of illness and jointly edited two collections of papers from the 1976 BSA Annual Conference and a reader on the sociology of nursing.

Gail Eaton Engaged in research at the Medical Sociology Research Centre, Swansea since 1973. Always concerned with drugs and their use; initially on drug information in general practice (with Peter Parish), now with Barbara Webb. Soon to be working on patient compliance. Has published various articles on prescribing in general practice.

Muir Gray Community Physician training with the Oxfordshire Area Health Authority. His main responsibilities are the problems of elderly people and the prevention of disease; he is a medical adviser to the City of Oxford on housing and environmental health. He has published books on self-care and care of elderly people.

Denis Gregory Research Officer, Trades Union Research Unit, Ruskin
College, Oxford (currently working with the Wales TUC). Employed
on research project jointly sponsored by the EEC and the Wales TUC
on the effectiveness and trade union response to interventionist
labour market policies. His publications include (ed.) *Work Organis-
ation; Swedish Experience British Context*, London: SSRC.
John Grigg Secretary, North Tees Community Health Council,
Stockton on Tees, Cleveland. Lecturer, Department of Industrial
Relations, University College Cardiff, 1974-1977.
Stuart Henry Sociologist at the Society For Co-operative Dwellings, and
also attached to the Outer Circle Policy Unit. He is author of *The
Hidden Economy* 1978 and co-author of *Self-help and Health* 1977.
His research interests include: part-time crime, self-help, co-operative
activity, community justice and workers' courts.
Margaret Miers Part-time tutor for the Open University. Lecturer in
Sociology, Polytechnic of Wales, 1974-1977. Research interests
include the sociology of medical knowledge, preventive medicine
and the professions.
Anne Murcott Lecturer in Sociology, University College Cardiff. Author
(with Margaret Stacey, Eric Batstone and Colin Bell) of *Power,
Persistence and Change* RKP 1975. Current interests include the
sociology of work and occupations, diet and health. Convenor, BSA
Medical Sociology Group 1979-.
David Robinson Senior Lecturer in Sociology at the Institute of
Psychiatry, University of London. Author of nine books on aspects
of medical sociology and the addictions and regular consultant to the
WHO Division of Mental Health.
Jane Taylor Lecturer, Loughborough University, Department of Social
Sciences, teaching social policy and administration. Her research
interests include planning in health services. Currently working on
research project on Joint Planning, on women and social security
and on comparative material on health services in socialist countries.
Barbara Webb Engaged in research at the Medical Sociology Research
Centre, Swansea since 1971, primarily in doctor-patient interaction
in general practice (with G. Stimson) and the present work on
clinical pharmacy and clinical pharmacology (with G. Eaton).
Publications include *Going to See the Doctor* 1975 (with G. Stimson).

AUTHOR INDEX

215

SUBJECT INDEX